PEOPLE, MEDICINE & MONEY

A Surgeon's Memoir

PEOPLE, MEDICINE & MONEY

A Surgeon's Memoir

JOHN C. GAISFORD, MD FACS

WORD ASSOCIATION PUBLISHERS
www.wordassociation.com
1.800.827.7903

Printed in the United States of America.

ISBN: 978-1-59571-448-0
Library of Congress Number: 2009936597

Designed and published by

Word Association Publishers
205 Fifth Avenue
Tarentum, Pennsylvania 15084

www.wordassociation.com
1.800.827.7903

|| TABLE OF CONTENTS

|| Introduction 7

1 || Pre-Medical School 9

2 || Vienna, Austria 19

3 || Georgetown Medical School 29

4 || Internship & Pediatric Surgical Residency 34

5 || Army—World War II 39

6 || People for People 57

7 || Back to the United States 65

8 || Resident—General Surgery—Pittsburgh 78

9 || Surgery & Money 87

10 || Interesting People & Companies 131

11 || People (Business & Golf) 161

12 || Surgery & Business (Home Care) 188

|| Epilogue 199

INTRODUCTION

Surgery is *medicine*, but in a variety of ways is a business. When one hears the word *business*, one immediately thinks about *money*.

The author has remained dedicated to the training and life of the surgeon. This book will make an effort to discuss medicine and money in a proper and honest fashion.

Surgery is defined in one dictionary as the branch of medicine that deals with the diagnosis and treatment of injury, deformity and disease by manual and instrumental means.

People will not have to be looked up in a dicti onary, but they will always be opinionated.

Business is "the occupation, work, or trade in which a person is engaged." Business pertains broadly to commercial, financial and industrial activity.

In this book, surgery and business will be observed in a variety of discussions. The word money will be noted in a somewhat questionable manner. But—isn't money interesting in many ways? Isn't money going to be of much more than just interest to many?

In the 1920s, 1930s and even the 1970s, money, people and medicine really did not create the problems that currently exist. However, medicine, people and business often are related and at times seriously related in some fashion for the betterment of one group or another.

1 || PRE-MEDICAL SCHOOL

Not every small town kid has an uncle who is a surgeon; I had Dr. Charles McGivern, originally from Kittanning, Pennsylvania (eighteen miles from my hometown of Chicora), who spent most of his surgical career in Atlantic City, New Jersey.

One visit from Dr. McGivern was especially memorable, as my uncle had brought with him a visitor. The visitor was Dr. Frantz Freml, head of the Department of Ear, Nose and Throat Surgery at the University of Vienna in Austria. Dr. Freml and my uncle became friends while my uncle was studying in Vienna under Dr. Freml. Little did I know at that time that Dr. Freml would really come into my life at a later date.

Listening to Dr. Freml and Dr. McGivern that day may have been the beginning of my interest in surgery.

The meeting with Dr. Freml and Dr. McGivern was during my last full summer in Chicora. Dr. Freml had been informed about the fact that I had always had a sincere interest in the German language, had taken two years of German in high school and two years of German at Kiski (learning to read and speak in

German). Dr. Freml rather promptly stated to me that should I ever be in Europe, his door in Vienna, Austria, was always open to me. Little did I have any idea about what would occur in the years to come – and that I would be working in the largest hospital – Allgemeines Krankenhaus – in Vienna, Austria. This position was obtained for me by Dr. Freml.

And now what could we do about college? My dad, a small town business man, obtained the name of a Pennsylvania state senator reputed to be in a position to assist those in his area in need of college financial aid, by arranging state scholarships. This senator, unbelievably, obtained my personal history from Kiski Prep School, where I was president of the graduating class of 1934 and honor roll for two years.

My dad and I were greatly surprised that we were granted the privilege of meeting personally with this state senator. We knew that there were a number of Pennsylvania colleges but had absolutely no knowledge of how to request our preference, even should a college scholarship be offered.

Our surprise was huge when this senator not only promptly offered me a college scholarship but suggested that I consider accepting as my college, the University of Pennsylvania, in Philadelphia. My surprise, of course, was overwhelming. Philadelphia was but fifty miles from Atlantic City, where my Uncle Charlie had his active surgical practice. That meant that without doubt, I could actually go to Atlantic City and possibly be guided in my decision to consider medical school.

There was no doubt in my mind at that specific time, that I would enlist at the University of Pennsylvania and attempt to be accepted into the premedical school division. My plan was that I would make every effort to graduate from medical school and become a surgeon. And what did this University of Pennsylvania scholarship mean financially? – a complete four-year scholarship, where the tuition was 800 dollars a year.

And so, I became a member of the pre-medical class at the University of Pennsylvania.

For quite awhile, many of my classmates remained quiet about what they planned to attempt to do in their four years at the University of Pennsylvania. Most of these students insisted upon being involved in classes about cat anatomy, anatomy in general, current medical and surgical techniques, and just about anything related to medicine. The thought among them was that having been involved in such a fashion, any subject related to medicine would improve their chances of getting into a medical school.

I just happened to disagree with most of my classmates. It was my understanding that at least the first year of medical school would be about the absolute basics relative to becoming a regular medical doctor—so why take subjects in pre-med school such as "cat anatomy"? Why not attempt to learn about subjects that would not be repeated in medical school and allow medical school to teach medical subjects?

My choice of college subjects included American History, English History, Philosophy, German speaking and reading classes and a few other non-medically oriented subjects. Approval was granted for me to take this work but that was not all. Luck was on my side again.

It took but a short amount of time to find out about the various departments at the University of Pennsylvania and one huge section, almost a college within a college, was The Wharton School of Banking and Finance. A trip to the proper section regarding the planning of my pre-medical school itinerary was quite successful. I requested to be accepted into the Wharton School but would remain in pre-med, even though

I would be majoring in English. This was approved and I then was on paper to take the following subjects over several years at the Wharton School: banking, economics, marketing and several others.

While I was frequently criticized regarding my choice of so-called pre-medical school subjects, it later proved to be an extremely fortunate college education. Later, in medical school, I didn't repeat any pre-medical school subjects. My educational choices helped me unbelievably in the beginning of a medical career.

At this point, I was still attempting to make a few dollars and help to pay my expenses. Financial help from home was extremely limited, but I did send my laundry home twice a month in a well-worn plastic box, and I was careful not to wear a clean shirt every day. The money had to come from somewhere to pay for room, board, transportation and extras. Odd jobs were just that – odd. The only connection one piece of work had to do with medicine was an interesting period spent at Thomas Jefferson Hospital in downtown Philadelphia. The work was not all that interesting. My involvement was checking pre-published medical papers and books for grammatical errors. My smartest decision in choosing subjects at Penn was becoming an English major.

There was one other piece of work that occupied my time off and on – playing in a college band. I had been taught how to play the drums and my xylophone when in grade school and high school and was lucky to be hired at Penn to play at times. This band – the "Pennsylvania Ambassadors" – was to be sold, as the owners were to graduate from college.

After some counting of pennies, I bought the band for about $300– a small fortune for me and I cannot recall where I ever found those three hundred dollars. Included with the ownership of the band was the task of contracting for jobs, providing transportation, paying the band, and keeping up with the modern music. Occasionally, a fraternity or other group for whom we played did not pay me, which meant that the members of the band were paid out of my own pocket.

For me, this no-account college band was business in every way. Business to make money to pay for food, money to help me pay my rent, money to rent one or two cars to drive to wherever my new band was to work, money to pay bus fare to and from Atlantic City to work with my Uncle Charlie in the operating room (and entertain thoughts about going to medical school later). For me, money just "kept me in business." And then in some way, a new on-and-off job appeared for me and my new band.

Not every weekend was spent playing at some kind of a party or dance. Not infrequently my doctor-Uncle Charlie wished for me to take the bus to Atlantic City where he had arranged a Saturday surgical schedule, which would mean that I would be his operating room helper. Certainly, surgical rules were quite different then, compared to 2009 medical regulations.

But my eyes were opened rather widely one weekend. Dr. McGivern's wife, Lee, was a beautiful woman and a good cook. She also had some extremely well-known friends. Some years earlier, she had shared living quarters in the East End of Pittsburgh with the best known actress in the United States, Lillian Russell. I never met Miss Russell, born in 1860, but I got to know her sister, Susie Allan, quite well. Susie was born in 1862 and had become a well-known actress in her own right. Miss Russell and Susie Allan were born within walking distance of The Western Pennsylvania Hospital of Pittsburgh, which hospital still exists there today. Both sisters were buried in Allegheny Cemetery, located one city block from The Western Pennsylvania Hospital.

Susie also was a close friend of the McGiverns' and stayed with them for several weeks in 1935. Because Susie was slim and small-breasted in her early life, her breasts had been markedly enlarged surgically about 1880 by having melted white paraffin wax inserted via syringe under the existing breast tissue. This was not an unusual technique in that era, but post-operative complications were not unusual either. Susie's complaint was severe pain, which was difficult to control with medications and without a doubt anyone in close contact with Susie knew that she was truly suffering.

So what was going to be done about all of this pain, the result of having melted wax injected under her breasts just to make her look more attractive to the audiences who viewed her stage appearances? Dr. McGivern and I removed both of Susie's breasts one morning. This obviously extensive surgery to remove the breasts of a previously internationally known "young" woman made her immediately more comfortable. And she was no longer a stage performer at this rather "old" age of 73 years.

At this particular time, anyone reading any of this story about having liquid wax injected into the underside of small breasts, not to make the breasts larger, but just to make them appear normal, would just toss this reading material aside. But why should one even think that this surgery was reasonable in any way? This procedure would not make any sense to an older person and how could this "older person" have any knowledge about more recent breast implants? A specific discussion will follow regarding breast implants.

First, another short discussion about the injection of liquid wax into the human body. Back in the 1940s and 1950s, it was not rare for a patient to appear at the Pittsburgh Presbyterian Hospital Clinic or my office with the complaint of having had liquid wax injected into the nose, eyelids, chin, or whatever—even the penis. However, the patient may have had complaints about pain, infection, or that the area which had been injected with liquid wax did not have the result that had been anticipated and well paid for. Many times, the injected wax had shifted its location, resulting in unacceptable appearances. In addition, this patient may have been having pain because the injected wax had shifted, as it changed its shape and rested against a nerve, resulting in pain.

In the early sixties (1964), a small group of plastic surgeons and one non-medical man met one evening in Houston, Texas. This group included Dr. Tom Cronin of Houston, now deceased; Dr. Robert MacCormick, professor of surgery at the University of Rochester, New York; Dr. Tom Reese, professor of surgery at New York University; Dr. Milton Edgerton, professor of surgery at Johns Hopkins University; Mr. Silas Braley, a representative of Dow-Corning Corporation, whose home was Pittsburgh, Pennsylvania; and me. The purpose of this meeting was to discuss whether or not it might be reasonable to use silicone prostheses to enlarge or reconstruct the female breast. Silicone was a Dow-Corning product. The decision that night was that Cronin, Edgerton and Reese would operate on a few chosen candidates and then we would meet and discuss the results. A number of cases were completed, but the initial plan was not followed.

Word quickly got around about this silicone procedure and Dow-Corning immediately supplied the requested implants. There was never a second meeting of this group. Many years later, the question arose as to why basic clinical research was not carried out to determine the safety of implanting silicone in the human body. The answer is quite clear. While the FDA (Food and Drug Administration) currently determines the right to use new surgical products, called devices, the FDA did not have this authoritative control until March 1984. Currently, countless numbers of medico-legal problems are costing millions of dollars. My cosmetic surgery interests never involved breast augmentative techniques, so my involvement with these implants was nil.

Our new job was quite unique. It had been offered to my band in some way but it's not possible to recall how it came about. Regardless – it was a different and educational piece of work for the "Pennsylvania Ambassadors." And where was this new job? At the Black Cat Inn.

The Black Cat Inn was a place all by itself, in a huge wooden building. It existed near a well-traveled road between Philadelphia and Wilmington Delaware, but was in New Jersey. It was extremely popular and the greatest bands in the country played there with regularity, having some unknown type of arrangement.

My band at the Black Cat Inn worked there in a somewhat strange and disconnected fashion, but we all liked our job. My band played the intermission when the real band members went to the bar or bathroom.

I became friendly with Kay Kyser and most members of his great band, including Ginny Simms. When I spoke with Kay Kyser, I always addressed him as Mr. Kyser and he remained a helpful friend for some time and would regularly send to me the stock band music (free) which publishing houses made available to him. We did not become closely friendly with any of the bands other than Mr. Kyser's group, but every band with which we were associated worked with us on a most acceptable basis. It was always first names in both directions. We met a number of these bands over many months, but we all felt that we would liked to have met them all. It was a great bunch of evenings for us – not hard work.

All of those college guys who played in the various bands, such as mine, knew that various ship lines were interested in these college music groups. For this specific reason, in some way, we contacted the United States Line which routinely offered these positions. Undoubtedly, the "evolving" history of my band, the Pennsylvania Ambassadors, meant something to the individuals managing the United States Line because we were promptly offered a position. And what was this job? On the tourist section of the President Harding, a 14,000-ton tourist class ship that traveled back and forth to and from Europe.

This came as a complete surprise to me, but arrangements were accomplished in no time. There would be no money paid to us, but tips generally were quite satisfactory to these college band individuals. A room on the ship would be assigned to the band individuals and we would eat with the passengers in the main dining room: the tourist dining room, of course. The timing for our trip to Europe was quite acceptable to me, but the other five band members had to be available. Because each member knew that I was talking with the steamship line, each was promptly apprised of the timing and accepted. Each knew when we would leave New York and when we would return and from which country.

We left New York on the President Harding in June of 1935. This 14,000-ton ship was rather small and couldn't handle high seas well. Seasickness among the passengers and our group was common. We didn't work very hard as working was impossible at times. Nonetheless, we reached England without major problems and our evaluation of that country was quite interesting. Some of the boys left London to see smaller towns, but I elected to remain in the city. My sightseeing consisted of taking a bus or trolley to the city limits and then struggling to walk back to the hotel where I would be staying. In London, I was within two squares of Piccadilly Circus, a most unusual area. At that time, hotels in Paris and London were cheap. I never paid more than three dollars a night and when hotels were difficult to locate at the price we were willing to pay, there were innumerable private homes where one could stay for bed and breakfast, and the price was many times less than two dollars.

London was never very interesting for me, even though my father's father and many of my relatives were from England.

Our return from England was uneventful and the weather in New York was good. I had a cousin who was an artist living in an apartment on 9th Street in Greenwich Village. Earle McGivern, daughter of my aunt in Atlantic City, was living above a Greek restaurant with a rather well-known young lady, Diane Barrymore. Diane was the granddaughter of the famous movie star, John Barrymore, and an actress herself. I moved in with them simply because there was an empty bed in the apartment. I had no money and the location was perfect for my going to and coming from England. My mother eventually found out about this arrangement, but it was never discussed – I just let her be a little concerned.

2 || VIENNA, AUSTRIA

That summer went quickly and school was again upon us. The work continued to be extremely interesting but difficult — particularly advanced chemistry, physics and mathematics (calculus being the worst!). I continued taking German, this being my fifth year with it. The medical students and physicians were expected to be at least capable of reading German because much of the medical writing originated in Germanic countries. I thoroughly liked German and with my three excellent years of German at Chicora and Kiski, I became fluent in conversational German – soon to be most useful.

It's rather hard to imagine why young college students, who had worked on an ocean liner to and from Europe, would like to try such a trip again. But all college students are not really smart and have not found a way to prevent becoming seasick. For some reason, I had some kind of a thought for wishing to work on another ocean ship and presented myself at the Cunard Line office in downtown Philadelphia one day, seeking information about a college band that was interested in a European trip. It was a great surprise for me to be informed that this huge British shipping company honestly needed college band groups who were interested and who had had previous experience with a ship company. It took but a few moments for this Cunard representative to scan the material I had available, which discussed the experiences my band had had with the American President Harding ship and a nice note from the American company for which we had worked in 1934.

In a matter of minutes, I arranged for my band, the American Ambassadors, to work on the Cunard liner, Georgic, in the early summer of 1936. All that I had to do then was to inform the members of my band that we had a job with the Cunard Line in the summer, June of 1936.

And so what transpired? The members of my band jumped at the opportunity of working on a Europe-bound ship again and were honestly shocked at the fact that I had signed an agreement to work on the absolutely gorgeous huge Cunard Line ship, Georgic. Our duties as a college band were quite carefully spelled out. We would play for approximately one hour before lunch, another hour mid-afternoon, and usually a third hour near the dinner period. We were requested by the ship's personnel to be available as "companions" for the college girls who might like some "opposite sex" dates. The number of such available college women was endless and we did our best to help the Cunard Lines.

As noted earlier, my uncle, Dr. McGivern, had done a large amount of his training in ear, nose and throat surgery in Vienna, under Dr. Frantz Freml. The surgical instruments Dr. McGivern had used for years in Atlantic City needed to be replaced and he then had an opportunity to obtain identical new ones – previously made by a Mr. Carl Reiner in Vienna. As I then was going to Europe again, arrangements had been made by Dr. Freml for me to work at his hospital that summer. New instruments that would be made for Dr. McGivern by Mr. Reiner would be delivered to Dr. McGivern when I returned to the U.S.A. at the end of the summer.

Dr. McGivern actually knew more about what would happen to me in Vienna than I. He and Dr. Freml probably had discussed a variety of things I would be asked to do when I eventually reached Vienna – I really was in the dark. There is no doubt that Dr. McGivern obviously personally felt that he owed Dr. Freml for what Dr. Freml had done for him previously in Vienna.

Europe and the United States were totally and completely different in 1936. But what could Dr. McGivern do for Dr. & Mrs. Freml? – a little but a lot! Dr. McGivern gave me six fountain pens to be given to Dr. Freml and eight pairs of nylon stockings for Mrs. Freml (nylon being absolutely unobtainable in Europe in the 1930s). But how to carry these terribly cheap – but expensive items through the various check points at country crossings? How could these so-called routine, relatively expensive but really hard-to-get items, get into Austria without being "caught"?

My Uncle Charlie was no dumbbell; he obviously knew exactly how the situation was to be managed. I was told exactly what to do. The six fountain pens were pinned specifically into the circular arm shoulder area of my personal jacket and Mrs. Freml's eight pairs of nylon stockings were securely sewn (sutured?) into the lining of the two sleeves of my raincoat by using rather larger-than-ordinary safety pins. One who has never traveled from one country to another will have to wonder why the pens and stockings were somewhat peculiarly placed, but at that particular time in almost every country, these items – pens and stockings – could cause the examiner of the in-country to check carefully and if the items were found, they could be removed from the owner and kept by the country worker who had discovered them. My stash of pens and stockings were safely transported from the United States to Austria.

Dr. McGivern gave me train fare to go from LeHavre, France to Vienna, Austria and then to Hamburg, Germany, where I would meet another Cunard ship for return to New York.

Dr. McGivern had told me exactly what to do immediately upon entering the city of Vienna: call Dr. Freml. How was I to know how to find a telephone? Where would I get the right kind of money to use a telephone? All kinds of thoughts ran through my head but I did make a sincere effort to watch my step when I crossed a street; traffic ran completely the opposite way from the United States as cars ran on the left side when going forward, not on the right side as they did back home. While I never got hit by a car, bus or cycle, I came mighty close a number of times.

It really was quite easy to reach Dr. Freml's office by telephone and I was informed to be at his office as soon as I could accomplish it, but after I had reached the Atlantic Hotel. The office staff in Dr. Freml's office had previously arranged for me to have a room at the Atlantic hotel, at $3.50 a day. Dr. Freml's staff also told me that a hospital working position had been obtained for me, at the Allgemeines Krankenhaus, within a city block of the Atlantic Hotel, and for me to report to Dr. Freml's office as soon as I could get there.

I had no difficulty in reaching the office of the Chief of Surgery of Ear, Nose and Throat – within two city blocks of the Atlantic Hotel and the Allgemeines Krankenhaus, the largest hospital in Europe.

Dr. Freml was a perfect gentleman and I remembered him readily as I had met him up in Chicora with my

Uncle Charlie a few years previously. He was somewhat surprised when I gave him the six new fountain pens from Uncle Charlie and the eight pairs of nylon stockings for his wife, from my Aunt Lee McGivern.

No time was lost in discussing the position that Dr. Freml had arranged for me at his hospital. The job fit perfectly into my previous medical training – I would be what could be known as an orderly, on a female surgical floor. It must be said at this time that I became an absolute expert at handling and emptying bedpans. But also, as a reminder, I was to be the one who would carry the surgical instruments being made in Vienna for my uncle in Atlantic City; instruments that for some reason had become somewhat shopworn; being only used on patients? These were the instruments that had been obtained by my uncle in Vienna and used in my uncle's office over the years in Atlantic City. Now, I was going to work all summer in Vienna and then cart all of these metal surgical instruments back to my uncle in Atlantic City (these tools were not that heavy). I have been told by the man who was in charge of having all of these surgical instruments made that if they had been sent to Dr. McGivern in some way, they would never have reached him – they would have been stolen and he, my uncle, would have had to pay for them and would never have received them.

Now that I was at work in this huge hospital in Vienna, I wanted specifically to learn all about the doctor whose extremely large picture hung on the wall in various parts of the hospital. This famous doctor was Ignax Phillipp Semmelweis, MD (1818-1865). He had been born in Buda, Austria, with that city later to become part of Pest, Hungary, and Pest then to become Budapest, Hungary. But why was this doctor so famous? Semmelweis proved beyond the shadow of a doubt that the proper use of water by doctors to wash their hands was mandatory to prevent serious infections frequently leading to deaths among the patients being treated. Those most seriously treated improperly by poor hand washing were mothers-to-be.

Many pregnant women preferred to have their babies at home because it was known that many died having their babies at the hospitals. The cause of death of these women in the hospital was puerperal fever or child-bed fever. Dr. Semmelweis showed that many medical students training at his hospital just briefly washed their hands before examining patients after working in the room where cadavers were being dissected, and transferred many infections to these mothers-to-be.

Dr. Semmelweis enforced the rule that anyone who was to deliver a baby had to thoroughly wash his hands in chlorinated lime before he even examined the patient. This technique reduced the death rate at this hospital from 12.24 percent to 1.27 percent in two years. Many doctors did not go along with Dr. Semmelweis, so he left this hospital and joined the University of Pest Hospital, in Pest, Austria, and became professor of obstetrics there in 1850. During his time there, he reduced the maternal mortality rate due to puerperal fever to 0.85 percent. This great work, as previously noted, was not accepted by numerous doctors of medicine. And then Dr. Semmelweis died in 1865, of a hand infection caused by a cut. He died at age 47 years.

There will be considerably more discussion regarding "hand washing" in the chapters to follow.

It is extremely easy for one to wash his hands casually, even though he may be about to examine a patient, or change the dressing on a wound. He may have forgotten about using water properly on his hands so that what is done regarding the patient is forgotten at that particular time. But that particular time of forgetfulness could result in an unnecessary problem for that patient.

The use of alcohol-based hand cleaning instruments (sanitizers) may result in excellent results in preventing infections – when they are properly used. Is the most important reason for the widespread advertising and selling of these alcohol-based hand washing machines to improve the management of patient's problems, or could it be to sell these products to make money?

Back to Vienna, Austria! This would be my home for the entire summer, so I had unlimited opportunities to see the city. And then I was just plain lucky – I met a medical student at the Vienna hospital where I had begun to work. This young man was really interesting. We hit it off promptly, and of course talking completely in German as my new friend knew no English. He was quite knowledgeable and sincerely interested in hearing about medical schools and universities in the United States. While I could not elucidate extensively on medical schools, we discussed colleges and the United States endlessly. My new friend's name – Mark Olander: and from then on I called him "Mark" and never had the necessity of coming up with his last name.

Mark was a great guide and we spent numerous hours, nearly always at night as he was in school and I was working in the hospital, walking the streets. We, of course, had no money for other types of transportation and only visited areas that were free. I still believe that the way for a beginner to see a city that one is genuinely interested in, is to obtain a city map and spend an adequate amount of time walking. And Mark and I really walked! He knew that city extremely well and made every single one of our numerous ventures outstanding.

One night we made an unusual walk, as we ended up at the Prater, the city amusement park – and it was free! It was a fascinating place. There was, however, one thing that could be done but it was not free to experience. This was the largest Ferris wheel in the world that we could ride on once for about twenty-five cents. It was stated that one seat could hold 25 adults or, as their brochure stated, six horses. We rode it once – that was enough. And then I shocked Mark, as I had previously been given information about the Ferris Wheel, that this wheel had been constructed in Pittsburgh, Pennsylvania, and that the name Ferris was a name that was extremely well known there.

Only once did I venture outside of the city. One beautiful weekend, I decided to hitch hike to Budapest, about twenty-five miles from Vienna, but in another country – Hungary. I didn't even consider the difficulty of entering another country, and I just assumed that people from Budapest, Hungary, spoke the same language that all spoke in Vienna, Austria (German). One does make mistakes once in awhile – and I made another mistake – mistakes that for some reason, I later made in medicine and surgery. In other words, I was an expert on making mistakes.

I was hungry. I had loose change in Austrian money but not any money that would be acceptable in Hungary. So – what to do? I did just exactly what made sense. I walked back across that river whose name I had forgotten, back across that bridge from Hungary into Austria – just across a handful of steps from one country into another.

I had no problem getting a free hitch hiker's ride back to Vienna – and I got some food!

And what did I learn in Vienna, at that great hospital? I learned a story about hand washing and surgery that too many doctors today should know more about. How many people die every year in the United States who may not have died if doctors, nurses and those caring for sick or injured people had properly washed their hands. One should just know how to properly keep his hands clean by using soap and water. What about the small box on the wall that is so often used to clean hands? It's O.K. if properly used but cannot beat soap and water.

The day that I knew I was to leave Vienna was to most people of Vienna a beautiful day, but to me it was just plain miserable. I loved Vienna, the great hospital in which I had worked, the medical work information that had continuously seeped through to nurses, doctors, and everyone regarding why everyone should learn why it was mandatory to wash hands properly.

The weather continued to stay perfect as I reached New York. The band members all were gentleman and issued many thanks to various individuals who worked on the Georgic. These ship workers even got through customs; please don't try to ask any of us how they did it, but our various musical instruments were not checked, nor our coats, not even the bag of surgical instruments over my shoulder. Come to think about it, none of us were even asked for our passports.

My personal story in New York was quite brief. I did stay one night at my cousin Earle's apartment on 9th Street in the Village. My financial status was not too bad; I had left New York for Europe with $75 in my pocket, spent most of the summer in Europe, and still had train fare from New York to Pittsburgh at the near end of that summer.

It was my fourth year at the University of Pennsylvania and I had applied to several medical schools. Several schools had accepted my application and had offered me the first year in medical school. Those that accepted me were Magill in Canada, Duke in North Carolina, Jefferson in Philadelphia; but the University of Pittsburgh?—no answer. But through an unbelievable game of golf one Sunday with the Professor of Medicine at Georgetown University School of Medicine in Washington, D.C., a great thing happened for me.

My golfing friend was Dr. Howard Strine, from Washington, D.C. His daughter was well known by my close relatives in Atlantic City, New Jersey and Dr. Strine had known that I was interested in medical schools. Dr. Strine talked with me in a sincere fashion, over a couple of hours, and then specifically asked me if I would be interested in going to Georgetown Medical School. When I sincerely gave him my obviously honest "yes," he said quite promptly, "You're in." Georgetown University School of Medicine was my medical school from 1938 to 1942.

Incidentally, that was the only day I played golf in four years at Washington, D.C., Georgetown University School of Medicine.

Back to my discussion with Dr. Strine. Dr. Strine knew absolutely nothing about my last years at the University of Pennsylvania. He had no knowledge of my college grades nor past history. We had not even discussed my previous interest in other medical schools. Things like this just happened – in some way. People just did good things for other people. Money was often not involved.

3 || GEORGETOWN MEDICAL SCHOOL

The first year of medical school was extremely difficult, with 100% being bookwork. Anatomy laboratory was three days a week from 1:00 to 5:00 PM, which included one hour of lecture followed by three hours of dissection of a cadaver. My two partners were hard workers and we alternated with the dissection. I might say that we had to take excellent care of that corpse (it was a he) to make it last nine months. He had to be carefully sprinkled with a proper preservative every evening (before dinner) and covered with a proper drape to prevent deterioration (and in the 1930s there was no air conditioning).

After the first year, medical school became considerably more like medicine – we began to see an occasional patient in "medical diagnoses" at Georgetown University Hospital. Even though school was a seven-days-a-week grind, just the fact that we would be seeing live people increased the interest for all of us. There was absolutely no social life and there were no medical fraternities.

Our third year became much more like what we thought it should be. All of our studies were related to patient involvement and we could see how eventually all of our night and weekend studying would have been worthwhile.

Obstetrics became a reality as we were sent out regularly to deliver babies. Occasionally two students went together, but frequently just one of us went. Transportation was a major problem and for weeks I went on my delivery cases by streetcar.

Early in the third year, it became necessary for me to find additional money to help pay tuition and all of the additional expenses associated with school. While my dad assured me that my yearly tuition would always be paid by him, I knew that family money was tight and so I was determined to find a job of some kind to try to help my dad. The yearly tuition was $800, which at that time was a huge amount of money. It must seem rather insignificant at the time of this writing, when the yearly tuition is about $42,500.

Room and board, books, transportation costs and incidental expenses were getting somewhat difficult to manage, but I was quite fortunate in securing work with Dr. Pete Moran. Dr. Moran was the Professor of Plastic Surgery at Georgetown. Internationally known for his outstanding abilities as a speaker, writer and innovator of difficult surgical operations, but not an important person to me at that time. He owned a rather large building in Washington, just two buildings from Dupont Circle. The first floor of the building with its opening at 2022 Q Street was rented by a general physician. This medical doctor was out of Washington at that particular time, serving in the Army for some reason unknown to me. Dr. Moran wanted to maintain this section of his building for this physician; I was told that rent would continue to be paid to Dr. Moran, and for these rather unusual reasons a quite unusual job was offered to me.

This job—and I was requested to find a classmate who could work with me—was so unusual that I accepted it promptly and told Dr. Moran that I was certain that I would find the proper classmate to work with me. Within three days, I found the right individual – Thadeus Nigborowicz. We lived together and worked together for two school years and we managed the practice of that family doctor in some fashion.

We were given one small room on the second floor of this old office building at 2022 Q Street. This room held a double decker bunk, one medium size regular office desk and one office chair. (The small room on the second floor was all that we had for two years). We could and did use everything that was available on the first floor, the office floor. There was a toilet, a hot and cold water sink in which to wash our hands, but no tub or shower. How did we wash ourselves? The medical school for some reason had a bathroom and shower, so for two years, Thad and I took a bath (once in awhile) at the medical school shower area. And we ate generally near our room off Q Street. A complete dinner at that time, in a common size restaurant, never exceeded sixty cents; and a tip generally was no more than ten cents.

Our "medical" coverage for this doctor's so-called medical practice was somewhat peculiar. We never wrote a prescription for any medicine, which would require legal coverage. We did write to request anything that anyone could walk into a drug store and purchase. We did use office equipment to look at a questionable fracture, using the same piece of equipment that was being used at that time in shoe stores, to check to determine whether or not a shoe was fitting a potential customer. In other words, we did numerous so-called “safe” things then that one would never consider doing today under any circumstances. What we really did was to save our dads a lot of money – and we both graduated with an M.D. from Georgetown Medical School.

After thinking about how we managed that medical doctor’s office, I shudder. We truly were completely honest in what we did but we could have gotten into unbelievable legal problems. And wasn’t this a piece of business? Wasn’t the combination of attempting to mold the obtaining of a medical degree with the obtaining of money to get that medical degree a combination of medicine and money?

During our fourth year at medical school, we had to make a plan regarding a medical internship. In October of 1941, I signed an agreement with an international fruit company to intern at a hospital in Hawaii. This hospital was involved in some business-like way with the fruit company. At that particular time, an intern there would be paid considerably more than interns in most American hospitals. This made me feel like a smart businessman. It is impossible for me to remember how this arrangement came about. However, my great plans were completely changed on December 7, 1941, when Japan attacked Pearl Harbor and the hospital in which I had planned to work was demolished. That made me start thinking about maybe how I could get into a Pittsburgh, Pennsylvania hospital after graduating in May from medical school.

Thad and I just kept working at 2022 Q Street and while Thad had already signed with a hospital in Pennsylvania regarding an internship, I just made a huge mistake after the Pearl Harbor Day disaster and let many weeks go by before I seriously thought about seeking an internship in a Pittsburgh hospital.

Obviously I was very late in looking, but I did communicate with Allegheny General, Mercy and

Presbyterian Hospitals. All were filled at that time but for some reason, Presbyterian Hospital could use one more. Even though the Presbyterian internship plan was for interns to work in pairs, I would be working without a partner. I accepted the arrangement and arrived at Presbyterian Hospital on July 1, 1942. That specific day, I was apprised that Presbyterian Hospital was called the Medical Center and the Center was comprised of Women's, Presbyterian, Eye & Ear, Children's and Magee Hospitals. The intern at Presbyterian would spend time at each of these hospitals, times being kept quiet.

4 || INTERNSHIP & PEDIATRIC SURGICAL RESIDENCY

At various times in this book on people, medicine, and money, money situations did occur. Some were of interest.

Interns were paid $10 a month plus room and board, but many months, I had money left over from my $10.

There were ways to make additional money if needed, and most of us took advantage of them. The most common was the selling of blood for transfusions. We could sell our blood ($25 a pint) as often as we could coax our blood-forming organs to produce more blood. Later, there became other ways to earn money and they will be described. Money always is creeping into the picture, whether the subject is surgery, golf, or business.

The rotation of the interns continued and my next one from Presbyterian was to Magee Hospital. I promptly learned how to deliver babies properly and enjoyed the relatively short period there. But everything at Magee was not about bringing babies into the world.

About that time, artificial insemination was being performed and Dr. Henry Irving, the senior resident in obstetrics at Magee Hospital, asked me if I would consider becoming a donor. The amount I would be paid was $25. After a check on that aspect of the business, I learned that Dr. Irving was to be paid $75 for each contributor he signed up, so I never became a nameless father.

As each week passed, more attendings left for the war. Having passed through several medical and surgical rotations, I was sent to Children's Hospital. The attraction the kids had for me was instantaneous and presumably my enthusiasm penetrated the observations of my staff people. Dr. George Foster, Chief of Surgery of the United States Steel Corporation (just having been Carnegie-Illinois Steel) and Chief of Surgery at The Western Pennsylvania Hospital, stunned me by offering me a residency in pediatric surgery – and not just a residency, but the Chief Resident position – and this after my being an intern for nine months. It would be nice to have thought that the position was made available to me because of my hard work and superior ability; but it was quite obvious that Dr. Foster and Children's Hospital needed immediate coverage for an exceptionally busy and undermanned facility. I immediately accepted Dr. Foster's offer and within a week, I was the new chief surgical resident at Children's Hospital.

As chief surgical resident at Children's my salary jumped to $25 a month and I moved into quarters at the end of the corridor on the 4th medical floor. (It may be of interest to learn that the chief surgical resident at Children's Hospital was paid $42,000 a year in 2009).

As resident surgeon at Children's Hospital, I remained in that position from April 1, 1943 until June 30, 1944 – a really long period in that busy job – 15 months!

Being a surgical resident at Children's Hospital was absolutely great. Every day was jammed with major problems. I was responsible for all surgery; general surgery, orthopedics, otolaryngology, trauma and plastic surgery. Since none of those specialty services had any residency coverage, I was it. The attending physicians on those services were glad to have me. They did not want to come in at night, be called for complications or take the time every doctor is called upon to spend when he is carrying on a busy practice. Most of the senior attendings in that era had a younger surgeon who was called an assistant, but the majority of the "assistants" were in the Armed Forces.

Very quickly the remaining surgeons "used" my availability and the "ability" they knew they had to have me develop, so that they, themselves could survive their drastically increased surgical work. An evening I will never forget saw my first abdominal operation absolutely on my own! A little Negro boy came in with an obvious acute appendix. It was clear, even to me, that he had to be operated on without delay. I called Dr. Evan Meredith, professor, elder statesman and to whose service the little boy was admitted. Dr. Meredith agreed during my call that the boy should be operated upon and he was scheduled for surgery, under general anesthesia, at 8:00 PM. When I asked Dr. Meredith what time he would be in, he said, "I'm not coming in!" – and it then finally sank in that I was to manage the case – my first, alone in that institution as "Chief Resident" (a position I'd held for all of 3 weeks). It wasn't exactly panic that set in, but I was more than a little concerned, although I knew I could open that abdomen and handle the problem. I called the new intern, whom I did not know, Dr. Henry Sherman. I told Dr. Sherman (later to run a very successful otolaryngological practice and remain a golfing friend to this day) that I had an appendectomy to do and that I had never done one. I asked him for his help. Henry said that he would be glad to help me, as he had never even seen an appendectomy!

The young lady anesthesiologist was well known to me and had superior talent. In addition, she knew that she could talk with and to me, so that she did not hold back any suggestions during the evening.

Henry and I set up a metal music stand, on which was placed a Gray's Anatomy book, opened to where the surgeon should be capable of locating the appendix.

The operation went along without any difficulty and everyone survived. Later, when I had time to really think about that first case, it was obvious to me that Dr. Meredith had not come in for a definite reason – he was helping me to grow up quickly in the operating room. He accomplished his plan, I think!

At one time during this Children's Hospital work, I thought that I could use a few more dollars. And I did not have "just a few more dollars" but a good friend, Dr. Francis Joseph O'Malley, an orthopedic surgeon at Children's Hospital and one of my teachers, came through with some help. He arranged for me to work two mornings a week at the Southern Wheel Steel Company in Homestead. Since I had no time off, except one weekend in fifteen months, the new job created a problem, but not an insurmountable one. I went to work at that job at 2:00 AM and worked until 4:00 or 5:00 AM. My job was to perform physical examinations on the men coming off the 2:00 AM shift, for which I was paid $5.00 per examination. For some reason, I was never caught out of the hospital. The night telephone operator was on my side and knew how to reach me should an emergency requiring my presence be brought in at the time I was at the plant in Homestead – and I never had a problem with cars I had to borrow to get to Homestead. (I owned none.)

There is no simple way to describe my fifteen months as a surgical resident at Children's Hospital. I ate and slept there – that is, when I found the time. Surgery occupied my time day and night for fifteen months – chests, abdomens, congenital problems, accidents, burns, fractures – everything! Many of my friends and colleagues questioned how I managed to get away at all to be married. Somehow I found a way. That residency at Children's Hospital in children's surgery was a great experience. And then the United States Army informed me that I was to report to Carlisle Barracks in Carlisle, Pennsylvania, on July 8, 1944. They had given me a week to go from surgery to the strenuous demands of basic training.

Many months previously, I had been plagued with bilateral leg thrombophlebitis, requiring hospitalization for several days. At that point, a physical exam by Army personnel prompted the Army doctors to inform me that the Armed Services would never accept me. Wishing to obtain training in adult surgery in addition to children (having been warned that one could not make a living managing surgery of children) a potential training position at the Leahy Clinic in Boston came to my attention. I promptly flew to Boston and was offered the position, which I accepted. True to Army arrangements, when I returned to Pittsburgh, I had orders to report to Carlisle, Pennsylvania, for basic training in the Army Medical Corps. I was in the Army!

The most important thing that happened to me during my lengthy fifteen months at Children's Hospital was when I married a wonderful young lady – Franny Jacobs. We have never had a problem between us and we are still together. At the time of this writing, she is 90 and I am 93. She was born January 18, 1919. I am ahead of her, having been born on June 11, 1915.

5 || ARMY—WORLD WAR II

The United States Army sent orders to me at Children's Hospital to report to Carlisle barracks in Carlisle, Pennsylvania, on July 8, 1944, to begin basic training. The report said that the training would be for entrance into the Army Medical Corps. At this point, Franny decided to quit her job and go with me to Carlisle. We managed to find a room with a couple of old maids near the post and my Army life began with no delay. The plans there were to give doctors a six week basic course and ship them anywhere they were needed.

A number of weeks went by at Carlisle as I learned how to crawl on my belly through mud under active overhead fire, scale walls, and slide down a landing net while carrying a full pack on my back. Why in this world would a doctor ever be exposed to such ridiculous experiences! None of this made sense to me in any way, though I would find myself in situations later on that made me change my mind. At the time, though, scaling a wall seemed hardly comparable to being called at 4:00 AM to offer an opinion about a baby just born with part of its brain exposed. I knew then that

that baby would have to have its brain area skin grafted within 24 hours so that it would not hemorrhage and bleed to death.

My weeks at Carlisle passed relatively quickly before my orders sent me to Camp Douglas, Utah. With my orders to go to Utah came more decisions. Franny decided to make the first move with me to Salt Lake, so on Army orders, we took a train west. Again, we found a place to live with no idea how long I would be in Utah. My stay there was less than three days, during which I performed general physical examinations. Orders then transferred me to Madigan General Hospital, twenty-odd miles from Tacoma, Washington.

Franny and I rented a trailer in the best place we could find – a rather run-down trail camp. Life in the trailer was fine for me but not very comfortable for Franny. I could shower at the hospital but the shower and toilet facilities at the trailer were down over a hill in a flimsy shack, with no lights and no wash basin–not like home.

My first day at Madigan General was somewhat unusual, as I took over a general surgery ward, which had lost its surgeons the day before. That day, I was told that I would do the surgical schedule the next day; which I did – five hernias. That was the first time that I had ever operated on adults. My anesthesiologist, Dr. John Bonica, was later to become one of the best known in the world in his specialty.

There wasn't much to be learned scientifically at Fort Lewis. Surgery consisted of routine work – innumerable hernias to repair, quite a continuing number of acute appendicitis cases and a smattering of odds and ends! This was to be expected, as most of the patients were young and most either being readied for overseas assignments or transferring to existing units in the States.

Dr. John Bonica and I became good friends quickly, a great benefit for me then and much more later. John later became a professor at the University of Washington. John seemed to take an interest in my having been trained in the surgery of children and in two weeks taught me many basic principles of anesthesiology. Little did I know at that time how useful this information would be for me – when I became chief of anesthesia of a hospital army unit at a later date in a strange country.

The weather was absolutely awful – for six months it rained daily, there was thick fog every morning, and penetrating cold. That Christmas was a unique experience in that I ate Christmas dinner with the professor of neurosurgery from the University of California in the large mess hall at the hospital. German prisoners were doing the cooking and while the food appeared to be quite good, it had been peppered with finely broken glass. (We finished Christmas dinner elsewhere.)

Things progressed rather routinely until I got my new army orders.

My orders? "Report to Camp Ellis, Illinois, December 29, 1944 (10-day delay en route) assigned to 92nd Field Hospital. December 20, 1944. Assigned as assistant chief of surgery and chief of anesthesiology."

My new assignment came as a shock. I had no idea what a field hospital was and only minimal knowledge about the functions of an anesthesiologist. And didn't it appear that I would be spending New Year's Eve at Camp Ellis?

My future was incalculable at that time. We promptly boarded a train in Tacoma for Pittsburgh. The weather in Pittsburgh was quite severe and I refused to buy an Army coat as I guessed I was headed for the Pacific and obviously hot weather. There wasn't a lot to do around Pittsburgh and Steubenville for a week except to wonder how long it would be until there would be a return trip. We never mentioned anything about the possibility of there being no return trip. Plans were made to communicate promptly about where I would go from Peoria.

I took the train to Peoria just before New Year's Day, 1944, and the weather was extremely cold, with heavy snow. My arrival at Camp Ellis was a rather different experience for me. There were thousands of men milling around, and no large buildings in which to house them. I was placed in the group, which was my field hospital group and new home. My "living quarters" was a small, non-insulated shack, which would contain about ten men. There was an old wood-burning stove but no wood, no water and that was it. I can't remember where we ate, or if we ate – I know very few had much of an appetite anyhow.

The next night was New Year's Eve, which again was meaningless. I did, however, have one good laugh. Out of some kind of a club came a familiar figure, Dr. Hank Irving, formerly chief resident in obstetrics at Magee Hospital. I could see him but he wasn't even seeing – I know he made it because years later he helped to deliver Linda, our first little girl.

Our stay at Camp Ellis was fortunately of short duration – about two days. We were told we would be leaving immediately for California, to go to Camp Roberts near Paso Robles. There we would be organized into a workable hospital unit, to be shipped somewhere into the Pacific area. (I knew about where California was, but I had no idea where or what Paso Robles was – a town, hospital, or something else?). I promptly called Franny to tell her what little any of us knew about our future plans and she decided with no hesitation that she would try to get to California in some way and try to find me. Her father (opposed to her plans) got her a seat on the El Capitan Train – to sit up for the 2½ day train ride to the West Coast. I'm still not quite certain how all of these quick plans jelled but Franny in some way found her way to Camp Roberts. Several other wives had maneuvered the same trip from various parts of the U.S.A. One was Pat Pool, wife of Dr. John (Major) Pool, chief of our hospital, and one who was to play a very important part in my life. Pat Pool and my wife Franny became close friends instantly.

Many lasting friendships were formed at Camp Roberts, as that was really the first time the hospital unit was a unit and we could actually see and meet the men who would be living together for a long time. Wives became friends and several trips to San Francisco during this period are still a real part of our past. John knew then that we would be shipped out of Pittsburg, California, on February 28, 1945. He quietly let me know about this February 28 date.

A daily conversation among us was "where are we going" and "when are we going." We knew we were to go to the Pacific. It remained important that there was no loose talk, particularly about troop movements—and John Pool and I took that problem very seriously. We were notified that we would be leaving California on February 28th and we had plans to drive to San Francisco on the 27th. John and Pat Pool and Franny and I drove up, but the girls did not know that this was our last night for an indefinite time. Women have always had that extra sixth sense of a change and, of course, they guessed correctly that we were leaving permanently in the morning as we were not returning to Camp Roberts but going directly to Camp Stoneman. I can still see Franny and Pat hanging out of the windows of the Stewart Hotel, waving goodbye but somewhat able to smile (a little).

We were quickly shunted onto the harbor boat "Catalina" to San Francisco harbor. Transfer of our entire hospital personnel – 20 doctors and 150 enlisted men plus all of our hospital equipment was to go to the U.S.A. T. Noordam. This was the largest ship owned by Holland and their greatest liner. Obviously, it had been re-equipped as anything but a luxury liner but it was a very fast ship. Because of the Noordam's speed, we were not to have the usual naval ships protecting us, even though we were carrying several thousand troops. (Several thousands or hundreds? How to know?)

I will always remember our first day on the water. We did not leave our dock until 7:00 PM and as we passed under the Golden Gate Bridge, the water immediately became choppy and I immediately became very sick. After a day in bed (and all the rooms were jammed with troops) and no food, I surfaced to find the weather warm and the ocean calm. At that point, I expected I would survive.

Not knowing what our destination might be, there was all kinds of guessing. On March 7, 1945, we passed within 100 miles of Hawaii – I don't know how that information came about. The ship was following an obvious zigzag course as we had a fast ship, not in a convoy and with no destroyers to ward off enemy submarines.

Sleeping was difficult. We were all packed tightly into stuffy cabins with multiple tiers in the metal bunks. All portholes were painted and heavily bolted for total blackout. There was no air conditioning and trying to find a sink or toilet not in use was a continual game. Because of the intense heat below, many slept on deck.

There was absolutely no information given to any of us. That is, I didn't hear about where we were and never heard a word about where we might be going. One strange situation existed and that was about the so-called 92nd Field Hospital personnel. Days went by before I even met the officer who had been assigned as the commanding officer of the 92nd: Major Howard T. Robertson, a general medical physician from Denver, Colorado. He turned out as a superior individual, a great leader, and a good helper as an assistant at the operating table – however, he was not a surgeon.

About once each day we would hear that we would soon see land and have to pack and be ready. But each day, we just heard that it would be the day that we would leave the ship – in what country? And then I had to return the typewriter that had been loaned to me. From then on, if I wished to make any notes, they would have to be written long hand.

On March 9, 1945, we crossed the equator and on March 13, 1945, we saw land – the island of Maliata, first in the string of the Solomon Islands. At this point, we heard we were going to Leyte. We passed Guadalcanal the same day and on March 18, 1945, we dropped anchor at Finschafen, in New Guinea – 6,000 miles from San Francisco.

We stopped at Hollandia in New Guinea, where there was a large group of ships, numbering about 50. The following day, we left New Guinea and had four naval destroyers as our protection, mostly against land-based Japanese airplanes. On March 28, 1945, we entered Leyte Harbor – and could not believe the ships there. We expected to leave the Noordam there as we were all packed. Plans were changed again and two days later, April 5, 1945, we left Leyte. On April 7th, we passed very close to the island of Corregidor; the Bataan Peninsula had no trees (all stripped by shells) and bomb craters were everywhere.

In a short time, we were again close to another shore and about 2:00 AM, we were again ordered to prepare to disembark. This was easy for officers (even for a lowly 1st Lieutenant such as I) as each man had to carry all of his possessions on his back, plus a rifle and a heavy cartridge belt. This type of hospital unit was the only larger unit where medical personnel were armed.

About 3:00 AM we left the ship, but not in the usual manner. We had to climb hand over hand down a landing net into landing barges and this under complete blackout conditions. The technique of net climbing was taught at Carlisle but I really didn't think that I would ever use that knowledge. The distance to the barges was the equivalent of going out of the fourth floor window of a building – and there would be no effort made to retrieve anyone should he fall into the water.

Once in the barges, we were on the shore in a few minutes, then were told to pile into huge trucks with no lights. One couldn't fall; bodies were too tightly packed. In about 30 minutes our truck bounced to a stop and our instructions were to dig a hole for ourselves and sleep in it. One of our young surgeons, Otto Brandt from Dallas, Texas, said, "I'm not digging a hole." At that point, a bomb landed with a tremendous crash (I thought it was beside me but it was probably a mile away). Otto started to dig so fast; I never knew where the shovel came from. I stumbled into what I thought was a bomb crater and being dead tired just put my head on my pack and went to sleep. In what seemed like 20 minutes, the sun awakened me, at which point I discovered that I had fallen into a sand bunker on a golf course (later I learned that we were on the Manila Country Club course and I have never minded getting into sand bunkers since that night).

On April 25, 1945, the 92nd Hospital and all individuals attached was moved 18 miles north of Manila, immediately adjacent to what was "called" an airstrip and used as one. Originally this so-called airstrip was an area on which the natives grew something.

On the very first day of operation, April 25, 1945, the 92nd was deluged with casualties, and we went to work immediately. Makeshift operating rooms were set up in large tents in a matter of minutes, not hours. Lights were quickly strung up at regular intervals above the operating tables, the power coming from dynamos that would also supply the heat to sterilize our instruments. Tents to house patients just appeared. The doctors, who were naturally more focused on surgery than on logistics, just assumed that beds would appear, and they did.

Almost immediately, boys with all kinds of war wounds were being brought in by jeep, ambulance, and truck; some even seemed to walk in on their own. How could such a thing be happening, not within days or hours but within minutes? My journal entry on that date said very little, I suppose because I was too shocked to be able to describe the real state of affairs. It is still terribly difficult to put it all down on paper.

We just did the best that we could do. At times, there were worse days but April 25, 1945 was our worst day up to that time – because as noted – that was our first day. It is still hard for me to believe how all of these non-medical guys could have possibly done such a great job of making it just possible for this bunch of doctors and nurses to work promptly with battle situations.

The 92nd was officially attached to the 6th Army and was supposed to be getting the injured from the 6th and 38th infantry divisions. And yet we would find that we could get patients from a certain army division on one day and patients from another on the next. We could never be sure which army unit we were working with, and it didn't make a particle of difference.

Initially, we thought it would be possible to single out and treat those with the worst wounds. But who was going to do this? John Pool and I were the only two medical physicians who had been trained to perform general surgery and abdominal work. John was the only one in the 92nd who was an expert in chest surgery. And I was the only one with any training in anesthesiology, however minimal it was.

And so, what did we do? We decided to string together three small tents to make one large operating room. This opened up the area quite well and allowed us to maintain some semblance of order. Each table area had its own set of instruments, depending upon the type of surgery it handled. We began to boil the instruments on one stove at the end of one of these tents. When we were satisfied that the instruments were sterile, we dumped them onto one big table. One man (obviously not a surgeon) was assigned to distribute the instruments as needed onto the various operating tables.

I was the only one who appeared to have a personal interest in the names of the many injured on whom we operated. I failed to realize that the administrative group spent all kinds of time attempting to keep records straight on these too many injured. Frequently we operated on boys whose names we never knew, and it didn't matter to us whether the injured was a major or a private.

We knew when we began caring for these wounded boys that we weren't going to save them all – but we tried, desperately, to the best of our abilities. In some instances, all we could do was ease their pain.

Maybe we couldn't change the destination of the train, but we'd try to make the journey as comfortable as possible.

Quote from a book or newspaper about the "journey."

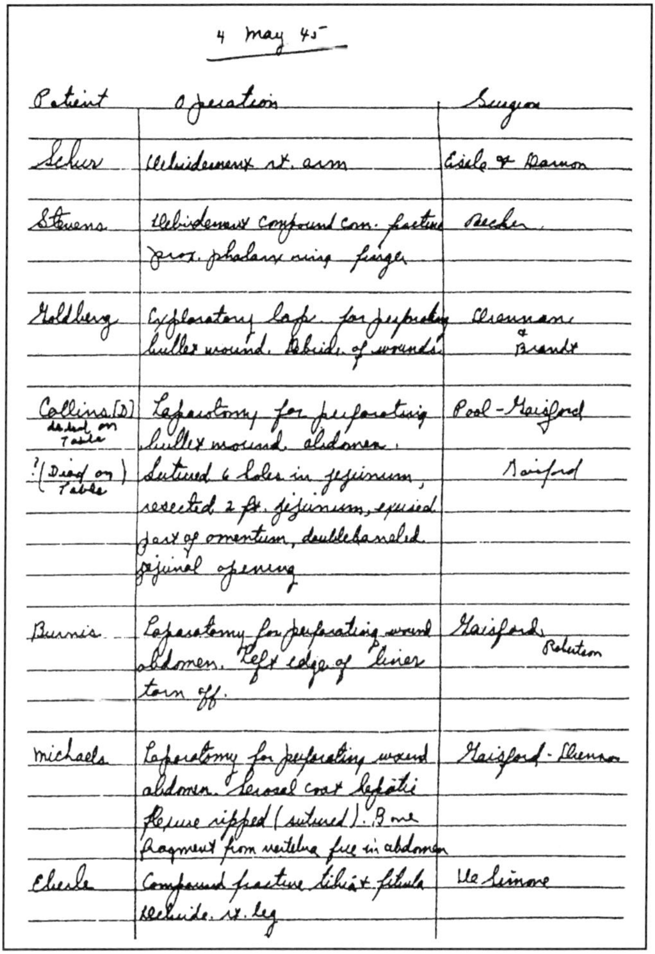

4 May 45

Patient	Operation	Surgeon
Schur	Debridement rt. arm	Eisele & Damon
Stevens	Debridement compound com. fracture prox. phalanx ring finger	Becker
Goldberg	Exploratory lap. for perforating bullet wound. Debride. of wounds	Ellerman & Brandt
Collins (D) died on Table	Laparotomy for perforating bullet wound abdomen.	Pool-Gaisford
? (Died on Table)	Sutured 6 holes in jejunum, resected 2 ft. jejunum, excised part of omentum, doublebarreled jejunal opening	Gaisford
Burris	Laparotomy for perforating wound abdomen. Left edge of liver torn off.	Gaisford, Robertson
Michaels	Laparotomy for perforating wound abdomen. Serosal coat hepatic flexure ripped (sutured). Bone fragment from vertebra free in abdomen	Gaisford-Ellerman
Cheale	Compound fracture tibia & fibula Debride. rt. leg	McGimore

JUST ABOUT THE BEGINNING OF SURGICAL WORK THAT WE WOULD BE FACED WITH—FOR HOW LONG?

After all kinds of surgery, the 92nd Field Hospital was split and a M*A*S*H Unit was formed. I was made chief of the M*A*S*H unit and ordered to go to Ballesteros, 400 miles north of Manila.

Several in this "Manila to Ballesteros" group were not positive about what a M*A*S*H unit was and "were we for sure one"?

This is an excellent time to describe a M*A*S*H unit. The 92nd had originally been set up much like a station hospital, larger than a field hospital but smaller than a general hospital. When the 92nd was informed that field hospitals were not used by Section (M*A*S*H) units in the vicinity of Luzon, many records and plans for reinventing itself were discarded. Now that the 92nd was about to dispatch a M*A*S*H unit after all, the necessary knowledge to do so was quickly reacquired, as the administrative staff had been oriented thoroughly to this type of operation while they were aboard ship.

The most specific information about the M*A*S*H hospital can be found in the magnificent book, Medics at War – Military Medicine from Colonial Times to the 21st Century. This book was written by John T. Greenwood, PhD, and F. Clifton Berry, Jr., and published in 2005.

The War Department created the 60-bed "Mobile Army Surgical Hospital," better known by its common name, M*A*S*H – a word formed from the first letters of each word. The War Department made the M*A*S*H absolutely official on August 23, 1945.

There will be more to say about M*A*S*H in the section on golf and business.

Of course, we did not know anything about the area through which we were driving. We had been given information about other hospital groups that we may see along the way, towns we may pass through, but none of this meant a thing to us. We would just keep driving.

So in 1945, I was in the center of World War II, chief of surgery and anesthesiology of a M*A*S*H Unit in the northern section of the Philippine Islands. And then – the war ended!

The 92nd Field Hospital

LATEST NEWS FLASHES AS COMPILED BY AACS

1300 15 AUGUST 1945

92D FLD HOSP
SECTION I

THE JAPANESE SURRENDERED UNCONDITIONALLY TONIGHT, TUESDAY AUGUST 14 AND HISTORY'S MOST DESTRUCTIVE WAR NOW IS OVER EXCEPT FOR THE FORMALITIES OF THE SIGNING OF SURRENDER DOCUMENTS AND CARRYING OUT THEIR TERMS. PRESIDENT TRUEMAN RELEASE STIRRING NEWS AT SEVEN O'CLOCK TUESDAY NIGHT, WASHINGTON TIME. WAR WEARY WORLD ALSO RECEIVED ANNOUNCEMENT SIMULTANE ULSY FROM MOSCOW, LONDON, AND CHUNGKING. ARRANGEMENTS STILL MUST BE MADE FOR THE SIGNING OF THE FORMAL SURRENDER TERMS. PRESIDENT TRUMAN SAID GENERAL DOUGLAS MAC ARTHUR HAS BEEN APPOINTED SUPREME ALLIED COMMANDER TO RECEIVE THE JAP SURRENDER. THEN V-J DAY WILL BE PROCLAIMED. THE PRESIDENT SAID,"MEANTIME, ALLIED ARMED FORCES HAVE BEEN ORDERED TO SUSPEND OFFENSIVE ACTION. " THE WIDE WORLD CELEBRATED WITH UNRESTRAINED JOY. PRESIDENTTRUMAN ORDERED THE JAP GOVERNMENT, WHICH ONCE HAD PROMISED TO DICATATE THE PEACE TERMS IN THE WHITE HOUSE, TO STOP THE WAR ON ALL FRONTS. THROUGH SECERATARY BYRNES AND THE SWISS LEGATION, MR TRUMAN DID THE DICTATING. HE DECREED THAT THE JAP GOVERNMENT; 1. DIRECT THE PROMPT CESSATION OF HOSTILITIES BY JAP FORCES. 2. NOTIFY GENERAL MAC ARTHUR OF EFFECTIVE DATE AND HOUR OF CESSATION AND SEND EMISSARIES TO THE GENERAL TO ARRANGE FORMAL SURRENDER. IN ADDITION, MR TRUMAN ANNOUNCED PLANS FOR SLACKING ARMY DRAFT CALLS FR 80,000 TO 50,000 PER MONTH. HE SAID THAT THE DRAFT WILL CONTINUE SINCE NOW THE QUESTION IS GETTING MEN WITH LONG, ARDUOUS OUT OF UNIFORM. THE DRAFT WILL CONTINUE TO PROVIDE REPLACEMENTSFOR VETERNS. THE PRESIDNET ALSO FORECAST THE RETURN OF FIVE MILLION TO FIVE AND ONE HALF MILLION SOLDIERS TO CIVILIAN LIFE WITHIN TWELVE TO EIGHTEEN MONTHS MR TRUMAN SUMMONED REPORTS TO THE WHITE HOUSE EXECUTIVE OFFICES TUESDAY AND READ THE STATEMENT WITH WHICH THE JAPANESE HAD REPLIED TO ALLIED SURRENDER DEMANDS. DAIS MR TRUMAN, " I DEEM THIS REPLY FULL ACCEPTANCE OF THE POTTSDAM DECLARATION WHICH SPECIFY THE UNCONDITIONAL SURRENDER OF JAPAN. IN REPLY THERE IS NO QUALIFICATION." THE PRESIDNET SAID THAT HE HAD BEEN INFORMED THAT EMPORER HIROHITO WAS PREPARED TO AUTHORIZE AND ENSURE SIGNATURE BY THE JAPANES GOVERNMENT AND THE JAPANESE IMPERIAL HEADQUARTERS TO THE NECESSARY TERMS FOR CARRYING OUT THE POTTSDAM DECLARATION. MR TRUMAN SAID ALSO THAT THE EMPORER WAS PREPARED TO ISSUE COMMANDS TO ALL THE JAPANESE MILITARY, NAVAL, AND AIR AUTHORITIES TO CEASE ACTIVE OPERATIONS.

THUS WAS THE SNEAK ATTACK ON PEARL HARBOUR FULLY AVENGED THREE YEARS, EIGHT MONTHS, AND SEVEN DAYS AFTER JAP PLANES STRUCK U.S. WITHOUT WARNING. JAPAN HAD PAID THE FULL PENALTY FOR THE TREACHERY THAT PLUNGED THE U.S. INTO A TWO FRONT WAR, THE COSTLIEST AND BLOODIEST CONFLICT. IN ALL HUMAN HISTORY. THE GREAT CONFLICT COST THE U.S. IN BLOOD AND TREASURE MORE THAN ONE MILLION CASUALTIES AND THREE HUNDRED BILLION DOLLARS. THE COST TO THE WORLD IS ESTIMATED AT MORE THAN FIFTY FIVE MILLION CASUALTIES AND ONE TRILLION DOLLARS IN MONEY, MATERIEL, AND RESOURCES. FOR JAPAN HAD MET THE END OF SAVAGE CONQUEST AND AGGRESSION, DISMEMBERMENT OF HER EMPIRE WON BY BLOOD SPILLING, AND DISARMAMENT AND OCCUPATION BY THE ALLIED POWERS. ONCE THE JAPANESE HAD STRETCHED FROM ATTUS TO TIMOR AND FROM JAVA TO INDIA. ONCE JAPAN KEPT A HALF BILLION PEOPLE ENSLAVED UNDER IRON RULE AND THREATENED TO ENFOLD ANOTHER HALF BILLION.

LATEST NEWS FLASHES AS COMPILED BY AACS

Ballesteros

NOW SHE IS DEFEATED WITHOUT INVASION, BUT AT TERRIFIC COST. FOR THE MOMENT, ALL THE WORLD FORGOT THE HORRORS OF THE CONFLICT WHICH HAD ITS START IN JAPAN'S GRAB OF MANCHURIA IN 1931. IN WASHINGTON AND THE REST OF THE NATION, SCREEMING WHOOPING, THRONGS LED OFF STEAM IN JOYOUS CELEBRATION. BUT OTHER THOUSANDS THRONGS TO THE NATION'S CHURCHES FOR PRAYER AND THANKSGIVING.

NOW THE NATION COMES UP AGAINST THE PROBLEM OF RECONSTRUCTION AND RECONVERSION, AND TO THE PERFECTING OF THE PLAN FOR PREVENTING SUCH CONFLICTS FROM AGAIN ENGULFING THE WORLD. PRESIDENT TRUMAN SPOKE ALONG THIS LINE IN AN EXTEMPORANEOUS ADDRESS TO THOUSANDS OF WASHINGTONIANS MASSED BEFORE THE WHITE HOUES. SAID THE PRESIDENT, " THIS IS A GREAT DAY. THIS IS THE DAY WE HAVE BEEN WAITING FOR SINCE DECEMBER 7TH, 1941 THIS IS THE DAY WHEN FACISM AND POLICE GOVERNMENT CEASES IN THE WORLD."

F I N I S H

** ** ** ** ** ** ** ** ** ** **

FROM HERE AND THERE WITH A LICK TO SPARE WISHING ENJOYMENT INSTEAD OF DISAPPOINTMENT I RESPECTFULLY SUBMIT- - -

THE NUMBER OF BABIES BORN TO MEN INTHE ARMED FORCES HAS EXCEEDED ALL EXPECTATIONS. THE SITUATION IS ESPECIALLY SERIOUS IN AREAS WHERE THERE IS A LARGE CONCENTRATION OF MEN IN THE SERVICE.

SAY DO YOU KNOW THEY HAVE A MILK STREET IN BOSTON? HE: NOW, WOULDN'T YOU THINK THEY WOULD HAVE FOUND AN UDDER NAME FOR IT?

LET FREEDOM RING

I'M HEARTILY IN ACCORD WITH THE CONGRESSIONAL RESOLUTION OFFERING IMMEDIATE INDEPENDENCE TO THE PHILIPPINES. HOWEVER, MAY I SUGGEST THAT WE AMERICANS BE GIVEN BACK OUR INDEPENDENCE AT THE SAME TIME?

All at once, we knew that Japan had surrendered. There wasn't much celebrating – some noise from a few guns and grenades. But the thing uppermost in everyone's mind was who would be discharged and who would get back home and *when*?

And then everyone began to wonder where we would be going. Invasion of Japan? Occupation of Japan? Home to U.S.A.?

The M*A*S*H Unit had previously received winter clothes – to wear when we "invaded" or now "occupied" Japan? Were we now actually in the 5th Amphibious Marine Corps as part of "Olympic Operation," the name given to the intended initial invasion of the Japanese mainland.

Specific orders were promptly received. The 92nd Field Hospital, with the Section I M*A*S*H Unit Ballesteros so-called hospital unit now reattached, would be shipped to Sasebo, Kyushu, Japan. This was almost the tip of Japan, but who cared? That is where the 92nd Field Hospital was going to go and we were going to work – work? – as a hospital in Sasebo, with a Marine unit hospital of some type.

What did the M*A*S*H unit do at this unbelievable time? It's hard to believe, but we still did some surgery, all of it on civilians. In addition, the one local medical Filipino, who had been mentioned earlier, was contacted again and we offered him all of our medical supplies and most of our scissors, knives and various forceps; to be picked up by him when we left the area – he was shocked but could not thank anyone enough.

And wasn't there a good chance that some may be sent to Japan, for some purpose? Like "occupation"? And wouldn't that keep certain ones from returning to the U.S.A.?

Major Clyde Drennan approached these various reports about Japan's surrender in a superior fashion. He sent the following notice to every individual in the unit.

HOSPITALIZATION SECTION 1
92ND FIELD HOSPITAL
BALLESTEROS LUZON
PHILLIPINES ISLANDS

18 August 1945

At 11:00 a short prayer service in commemoration of the war's end will be held.

HYMM: Onward Christian Solders
INVOCATION PRAYER: Pfc Angelo
A SHORT TALK BY MAJOR DRENNAN
THE STAR SPANGLED BANNER
(All Sing)

CLOSING PRAYER: One minute of silent prayer followed by The Lord's Prayer in unison

PRAISE GOD WHO HAS ALLOWED US TO EMERGE VICTORIOUS IN THIS WAR FOR HUMANITY.

Not one individual missed this prayer service. Of course we had no musical instruments but every single young guy joined in singing "Onward Christian Soldiers." Following this, Major Drennan asked Pfc (Private First Class) Angelo to give a prayer, which led to Major Drennan offering a superior talk about the end of the war. Following Major Drennan's talk, everyone sang the "Star Spangled Banner." The service ended with a minute of silent prayer and a quiet repetition of the The Lord's Prayer in unison.

Orders kept coming along. I was to be one of the 92nd who would be shipped to Sasebo and to be on a ship again was not in any way of interest to me.

Hq. 92d Fld Hosp, APO 929, Subj: Historical Report, 15 Aug to 30 Nov 45, dated 30 Dec 45.

The unit sailed for Japan on the USS Queens (AP 103) on 8 October 1945 and anchored in the harbor of Sasebo, Kyushu, Japan the morning of 13 October 1945, after a rough but uneventful trip. Supplies and equipment were unloaded by small craft to a shore dump site from 18 October to 24 October 1945. Upon completion of this, the personnel moved ashore, 25 October 1945, into the barracks of the former Japanese Naval Trades School in Sasebo.

On 13 November 1945, the 92d Field Hospital assumed control and operation of the Corps Evacuation Hospital No. 1, USMC, located in the Trades School Area, with a status of approximately 273 Army, Navy and Marine patients. From that date until 30 November 1945, the unit has continued to operate as a station hospital in furnishing the best possible medical service for the occupation forces in the Sasebo area.

The attitude of the Japanese people, as noticed by this command, has been one of mixed subservience, indifference and resentment. However, no overt acts of hostility have been made toward any member of this command, and Japanese workers employed in the hospital area have been cheerfully cooperative and good workers.

It is felt that the ability to be able to set up a hospital and handle a great variety of surgical and medical cases in a short time under peace-time occupation conditions as well as under field combat situations, demonstrates the adaptability and versatility of the modern Field Hospital.

FOR THE COMMANDING OFFICER:

H. M. STEWART
Captain, MAC
Adjutant

The army sent the following article to the 92nd Field Hospital, which article was then distributed to the 92nd and the attached M*A*S*H Unit.

The 92nd Field Hospital

THE OCCUPATION IS PROCEEDING WITH SMOOTHNESS THAT DISPATCHES DESCRIBE AS FANTASTIC. JAPANESE NEWSPAPER MEN STOOD SIDE BY SIDE WITH ALLIED CORRESPONDENTS FRIDAY AS IF THERE NEVER HAD BEEN PEARL HARBOR, WHILE GENERAL MAC ARTHUR GAVE HIS FIRST INTERVIEW IN JAPAN. MAC ARTHUR SAID "MELBOURNE TO TOKYO WAS A LONG, HARD, ROAD, BUT THIS LOOKS LIKE THE PAYOFF. THE SURRENDER PLAN IS GOING ON COMPLETELY ACCORDING TO PREVIOUS ARRANGEMENTS. IN OUTLYING THEATERS FIGHTING HAS PRACTICALLY CEASED. IN THIS AREA 300,000 JAPANESE TROOPS HAVE BEEN DISARMED AND DEMOBILIZED. THE JAPANESE SEEM TO BE ACTING IN COMPLETE GOOD FAITH AND THERE IS THE PROSPECT OF SUCCESS OF THE CAPITULATION WITHOUT UNDUE FRICTION AND WITHOUT UNNECESSARY BLOODSHED."

****

SMOOTH AS THE OCCUPATION IS, IT IS NOT BEING ACCOMPLISHED WITHOUT THE FIRING OF A SINGLE SHOT. SKYMASTERS CARRYING GENERALS EICHELBERGER AND SWIFT DREW A BURST OF ANTI-AIRCRAFT FIRE WHILE PASSING OVER AN ISLAND 80 MILES SOUTH OF YOKOSUKA. THE AIM WAS BAD BUT IN THE WORDS OF CAPTAIN J D HUTCHINSON OF SALIDA, COLORADO, "THE JAPANESE WERE DAMNED WELL SHOOTING AT US."

****

MEANWHILE, IN TOKYO BAY, MEDICS ARE BUSY EVACUATING THE FIRST CONTINGENT OF ALLIED WAR PRISONERS IN HOSPITAL SHIPS. THEY NUMBER MORE THAN 500, INCLUDING SOME OF THE WORLD'S OUTSTANDING HEROES. ONE OF THEM IS THE FAMOUS MARINE ACE, MAJOR GREGORY BOYINGTON. HE SAID HE WAS BEATEN WITH A BASBALL BAT BESIDES UNDERGOING OTHER FORMS OF MISTREATMENT. ALL LIBERATED PRISONERS TOLD OF HUNGER, PRIVATION, HUMILIATION, AND VARIOUS FORMS OF BRUTALITY.

****

ON THE OPPOSITE NOTE, TOKYO RADIO QUOTES A JAPANESE CORRESPONDENT AS WRITING THAT THE ENEMY GOVERNMENT SHOULD NOTE THE FRIENDLY ATTITUDE OF THE AMERICANS. THE WRITER SAID THE AMERICANS DO NOT REVEAL THE HAUGHTY ATTITUDE OF VICTORS.

STATESIDE:

IN THE UNITED STATES THE STATE DEPARTMENT HAS RELEASED A HITHERTO UNPUBLISHED LETTER BY FORMER SECRETARY OF STATE CORDELL HULL IN WHICH HULL FLATELY DENIES HE EVER ISSUED ANY ULTIMATUM TO THE JAPANESE BEFORE PEARL HARBOR. THE LETTER WAS WRITTEN BY HULL TO SECRETARY OF WAR STIMSON LAST SEPTEMBER 28 AND WAS RELEASED BY PRESENT SECRETARY OF STATE JAMES F BYRNES, APPARENTLY AS AN ANSWER TO THE CRITICISM OF HULL BY THE ARMY BOARD OF INQUIRY WHICH INVESTIGATED THE PEARL HARBOR DISASTER. HULL SAID THAT ON NOVEMBER 25 OF 1941, HE INDICATED THAT THE QUESTION OF THE COUNTRY'S NATIONAL DEFENSE FROM THAT POINT ON SHOULD BE ESPECIALLY THE CONCERN OF THE ARMY AND NAVY.

(continued)

****

MEANWHILE, PRESIDENT TRUMAN SAID HE HAD NO OBJECTION TO ANY COURTS MARTIAL ARISING FROM REPORTS OF THE PEARL HARBOR DISASTER, BUT HE SAID HE HAS NO INTENTION OF ASKING FOR THEM HIMSELF. THE PRESIDENT SAID HE THOUGHT THE COUNTRY AS A WHOLE WAS AS MUCH TO BLAME FOR THE PEARL HARBOR DISASTER AS ANY INDIVIDUAL.

****

A NEW YORK JUDGE TODAY HANDED DOWN A DECISION WHICH AFFECTS ALL VETERNS. FEDERAL JUDGE ABRUZZO DECLARED THAT A WORLD WAR II VETERAN WAS ENTITLED TO THE JOB HE HELD BEFORE ENTERING SERVICE, EVEN THOUGH REHIRING HIM MAY MEAN THE DISMISSAL OF A WORKER WHO HAS SENIORITY. THE DECISION WAS HANDE'D DOWN IN THE CASE OF A VETERAN REHIRED BY HIS FORMER EMPLOYER, BUT LATER DISMISSED. THE VETERAN WAS LET OUT WHEN WORK WAS SLACK BUT ANOTHER WORKER WHO WAS NOT A VETERAN WAS RETAINED. ACCORDING TO THE JUDGE THE VETERAN WAS ENTITLED TO PREFERANCE EVEN THOUGH HE HAD LESS SENIORITY.

F I N I S H

N A N C Y

HER NAME WAS NANCY,
SHE WAS ONE OF THE BEST,
LAST NIGHT I PUT HER TO THE TEST.

I LOOKED AT HER WITH GAY DELIGHT,
LORD, I KNEW SHE WAS MINE TONIGHT.

SHE LOOKED SO SWEET, SO PRETTY, SO SLIM,
THE NIGHT WAS DARK, THE LIGHT'S WERE DIM.
I WAS SO EXCITED MY HEART SKIPPED A BEAT,
BECAUSE I KNEW SHE WAS IN FOR A DARN GOOD TREAT.
I'D SEEN HER STRIPPED, I'D SEEN HER BARE,
I'D FELT HER OVER EVERYWHERE.
I GOT INSIDER HER ----
SHE SCREAMED WITH JOY - OH! BOY!
I GOT HER UP QUICKLY, AS QUICKLY AS I COULD,
I HANDLED HER GENTLY, FOR I KNEW SHE WAS GOOD.
I ROLLER HER OVER, THEN ON HER SIDE,
THEN ON HER BACK I ALSO TRIED.
SHE WAS JUST ONE THRILL, THE BEST IN THE LAND,
THAT FLYING FORTRESS OF THE 8TH BOMBER COMMAND...............

The separation of the Section I unit from the 92nd Field Hospital resulted in a lack of communication between the two. Certainly the officers in charge of each unit collaborated, but the medical personnel of the Ballesteros group had no knowledge of any plans involving both groups.

6 || PEOPLE FOR PEOPLE

Up to this point, I have not discussed the numerous great things that have been done for others without consideration for money. There is much to be discussed about great individuals and groups. Many pieces of interest will mix money and real help for people that at times involved multibillion dollar companies working to make money—but also helping people, in ways that will be described in various ways. And all of this great help for others was in many ways not about making money – even though there was a very close relationship between *money* and *people.*

Surgery for us in Sasebo was minimal as most medical problems, non-surgical, were managed by non-surgeons. However, there were numerous surgical and medical situations among the Japanese people in Sasebo. The 92nd was absolutely not permitted to admit or treat anyone outside of the American Armed Services.

There was no rule; however, about helping the locals outside of the American Hospital, so I made a visit to the Imperial Hospital of Sasebo.

There was only one person at this hospital—a nurse—who could speak English. I asked this young woman to find out if the director of surgery there had any interest in discussing surgery with me or needed surgical assistance of any kind. She disappeared into an office and about ten seconds later the director of surgery emerged. This surgeon – his name did not lend itself to be spoken by an American – was a true gentleman. Although he spoke no English, we were able to communicate in an almost normal manner, thanks to the help of the female translator. I learned that this hospital needed everything. I offered my services in everything for which I had been trained – all general surgery, except chest surgery.

Our partnership began promptly and continued during the entire period that the 92nd remained in Sasebo. Anesthetic equipment was minimal. Fortunately all anesthetics – spinal, intravenous, and local – were taken care of by the Japanese. There was no equipment for endotracheal anesthetics. (Tubing could be inserted into the trachea, and the patient put to sleep by intravenous or inhalation gas, with the anesthetist using normal pressure. Such a procedure would pose limitations for many types of lung or heart surgery.)

What was even more astounding than the lack of anesthetics was the complete lack of antibiotics of any kind. And there were no surgical gloves either. That meant that all surgery was performed barehanded. This was a sad state of affairs, but it had its rewards. On a somewhat daily basis, we performed surgery, ninety percent of it abdominal, and we employed every kind of procedure. At no time did I perform any surgery alone. The Japanese surgeon always had me as his assistant.

It is hard to believe that, given the lack of antibiotics and surgical gloves, there were few complications.

As I mentioned earlier, my training had been in pediatric surgery. At the time of my entrance into the 92nd Field Hospital, I had had very little experience with adult problems. Pediatric surgery requires the utmost care in the handling of tissues. Imagine the precision involved in touching, moving, cutting, and sewing the abdominal organs and skin of a day-old baby – all of this with appropriate coverage of anesthetics and the very best instruments. These surgical techniques were not new. Doctors showed great understanding of them a long time ago. Unfortunately, many of these techniques have been relegated to the back burner today.

While these statements regarding pediatric surgery could never be forgotten by one trained in the surgery of newborn babies, the technique of careful handling should be used by *all* surgeons. But today, too many mistakes regarding the use of soap and water are being made.

If the surgeon uses basic common sense, handling tissues with extreme gentility only after adequately washing the hands with soap and water, infection rates will be minimal for that surgeon's patients. As for surgical gloves, it is commonly known that gloves can be punctured during surgery or dressing changes, resulting in leakage. Doesn't it make sense that there would be fewer bacteria if hands were washed thoroughly before the gloves were put on?

This Japanese surgeon did more for the patients who needed his surgical care than any surgeon that I could picture. The Japanese nurse who could speak with me in English just told me, with tears in her eyes, that this doctor was going to kill himself working – day after day, night after night, occasional food and sleep – it was just more than I could imagine. None of this surgical work was for money. This doctor was just a plain surgical doctor —just helping the ones who needed his type of care. I learned many *good* things about surgery and people that I would never forget. And to repeat – *money* was never involved regarding surgical work. This surgeon worked just to help people who needed surgical help.

I learned a tremendous amount by working with this Japanese surgeon and I just hoped that I helped him and his patients – just by working with him. As mentioned, he was not only a superior surgeon; but he was not working for money. First of all, there just was no available money for Japanese hospital work of any kind. This surgeon worked countless hours - days and nights –for any Japanese individual who needed the type of care that he could offer.

I will never forget the day that I told the English-speaking nurse at the Japanese Imperial Hospital of Sasebo, Japan, that I was leaving.

This superior chief of surgery at this Japanese hospital was told by the English-speaking nurse that I was leaving that day – and, of course, we all knew that none of us would ever see one of the other again. The nurse told the Japanese surgeon that I was leaving – and – this wonderful Japanese doctor gave me a real tight, long, meaningful squeeze – and in some kind of word in English, attempted to thank me for working with him.

Could anyone ever forget such an experience? To me, this surgeon did a huge amount of surgical work for others, just because he was a down-to-earth great doctor.

This new friend, a great new friend, just said goodbye in an effort to say the word in a non-Japanese word, and gave me a second, thankful, real squeeze. Friends can be friends in a variety of ways.

Plans were then being made for the 92nd Field Hospital to join up with the 118th Station Hospital in

Fukuoka, a city of approximately 400,000 people, on Kyushu. From Fukuoka, maybe I would learn when and how I might get home.

The 92nd Field Hospital was in Fukuoka, Japan. Dr. John Pool, chief of surgery of the 92nd Hospital, and I as assistant chief of surgery of the 92nd, were now working with the 118th Station Hospital there in Fukuoka in 1945.

Surgery now that the war had ended was vastly different, being routine in just about anything. And so, John Pool and I did not have much surgery to perform. The chief of surgery of the 118th Station Hospital ran the surgical service. And so – what did John and I do?

I really had the answer as to what John Pool decided to do at that particular time. Having been second in command surgically with the 92nd, with John Pool first and great, I instantly agreed to what John said was going to be done. I was not asked, but told!

John Pool was feeling that he had too much time on his hands. And so did I. He came up with a plan. We would start a dog lab and he would teach me everything he knew about chest and abdominal surgery—all types of techniques. It was simple to plan our animal surgery hospital. An empty building next to the 118th Station Hospital proved to be the ideal setting for it. There were countless men around who had no money and no job, and as many dogs running wild in the area. It took very little time to hire help and to locate research subjects.

John Pool worked with me tirelessly. He had absolutely nothing to gain by spending many, many hours showing me how to remove a lung or part of a lung, or how to repair or remove segments of the intestinal tract. But I knew that in helping me, John was helping himself. He needed to work, and operating with me kept both of us reasonably sane. Sure, I had already been working on chests and abdomens for many months and I believed that my work had been acceptable. But I stood to learn a lot more with John Pool at my side, working on those dogs. Among other things, he taught me how to teach. I remembered those days with John with gratitude when I was in various teaching positions in the years that followed.

John Pool taught me in a surgical fashion, for which I could never have thanked him enough. A surgeon – teaching surgery!

Time didn't stand still, but it sure moved slowly. The days dragged by without incident—that is, until November 22, 1945, Thanksgiving Day. A group of Marines were sitting around some boxes of explosives when some of the explosives went off. Several of these boys were killed outright, but the ones who survived the initial blasts were brought to John Pool and me at the 118th. We operated immediately. Unfortunately, some died on the operating table. It was a bad Thanksgiving.

The month of December began on a much happier note. We got packages from home. John Pool and I received eleven boxes of food: anchovies, sardines, crackers, etc. – all kinds of small cans. We selected a few of the items for ourselves before we opened the door to anyone else who might have a desire for something from home. These cans of food were gone in no time.

On the twenty-fifth day of December, Christmas Day, John and I operated all day long on several very bad auto accident victims. This was our last day in the operating room together. There was a special dinner that night but John and I didn't go – we were too tired – and besides, we still had some things to eat that had come from New York and Pennsylvania.

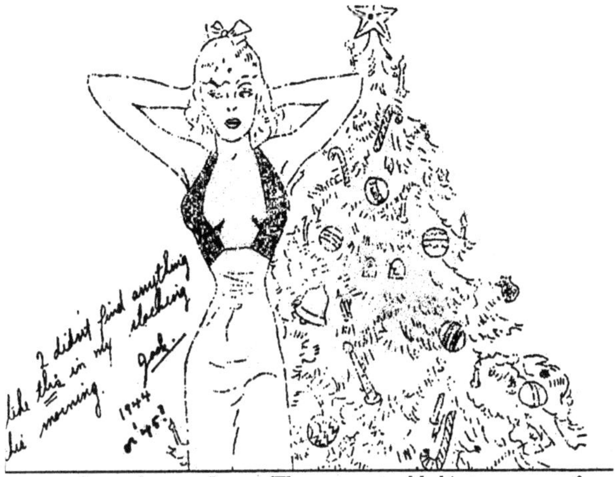
I didn't find anything
like this in my stocking
this morning. Jack.
1944
or '45?

Somewhere on Luzon (The comment added is true: no one from the 92nd found anything like this in Luzon on Christmas morning!)

THIS CHRISTMAS PICTURE WAS SENT TO MY WIFE.
SHE MAY STILL HAVE IT!

Crossing the Pacific Ocean this time was relatively comfortable and quick. We reached San Francisco harbor the morning of July 4, 1946. Of course, there were innumerable chores for the crew, but we as doctors expected to leave that ship within the hour. A rapid exit was not to be, as the union workers would not unload the ship on a holiday. That meant we would be forced to wait until July 5th. What a disappointment, not to be able to call home after waiting for two years!

I got on the ship with $75 and that 4th of July got into a poker game: table stakes, straight five-card draw. About 3:00 AM, I had improved my financial status about $700. The next hand I never forgot, being dealt three natural queens and with two people betting into me. When I drew two cards, one of which was a fourth queen, it became rather interesting – there were still bets into me. Finally, one boy at the table whom I had gotten to know and like, asked me how much money I had. When I counted out $750, he raised me $750. I called him and when he put down four nines, I was almost $2,000 richer. (That paid many bills in the ensuing months!) And then it was July 5th.

A follow-up on that is rather hard to believe. At the beginning of a court case in 1986, a nicely dressed man (the lawyer for the client I was appearing against – Herb Rosenberg - I learned his name years later) walked past and said to me, “Do you remember those four nines?” This was Herb Rosenberg, the man whose $750 I had separated from him in 1946.

Several years following this 1986 court case, another legal situation arose involving one of my burn cases. While I was just a witness for the burn patient, who had been my patient, my friend Herb was one of the lawyers for the patient. Herb, rather soon after that case became my personal lawyer, and never over the years, would allow me to pay him anything for the numerous hours he put in working professionally on my personal problems.

7 || BACK TO THE UNITED STATES!

NEW YORK PRESBYTERIAN HOSPITAL

In 1946 it was just great to be back in the United States. However, what was I capable of doing from a medical-surgical standpoint? What I really wanted to do was surgery, but my training in surgery was just army style. My ability in performing general surgery was minimal, regarding the earning of even an amount of money that would pay the bills to just eat and sleep.

The decision was made that I would attempt to find a hospital that would accept me as a surgical resident. I rented a car and drove to Philadelphia, Baltimore and Washington, visiting established hospitals that I knew had first-class surgical training programs. The result? Nothing available! And so, I went home: what to do?

While I was on my trip to the various cities and hospitals a telegram had arrived at Chicora for me – a telegram from Dr. John Pool. What did John say in his telegram to me? – that he had obtained a fellowship for me in the Department of Surgical Pathology under Dr. Arthur Purdy Stout. Did I want it? I called John the next day after I had read his telegram, to thank him for even thinking about me. It sounded to me as if this would fit into my "complicated" schedule. John told me that I would not be paid *anything* but that he thought that this fellowship would help me immensely.

Although John said that he would call Dr. Stout's office to tell them that I would accept the fellowship with Dr. Stout, it was my feeling that I should promptly go to New York and introduce myself to Dr. Stout. I left that night by train, arrived in New York early the next morning and took the subway train, in that long uptown ride, to a new place: 168th Street and Presbyterian Hospital.

I had no problem finding Dr. Stout's office; fortunately Dr. Stout was in and had the time to see me. I was instantly impressed by the ultra calm fashion in which Dr. Stout greeted me, just as if I held some kind of an important position in something.

Dr. Stout and I had a nice discussion about what chores I would have in my fellowship position and he briefly mentioned what he believed I might learn there. It was a most successful meeting; I promptly felt that I had made a really good decision to have accepted this fellowship.

My talk with Dr. Stout was brief but impressive. I left his office and the hospital to rather promptly catch a subway returning to the downtown train station. I was just plain lucky to find a train going to Pittsburgh within an hour and got home by late afternoon.

Franny and I discussed my having taken the position with Dr. Stout in New York. We agreed promptly that we should go to New York to live. But how could we live in New York?

Franny and I had done a lot of talking with each other on our seven-hour train ride to New York. We were quite aware of the fact that our financial situation was just plain bad. Had it been reasonable to accept a full time position, when the pay was going to be zero? And what was Franny going to do all day every day with nothing to do except maybe read books and newspapers or possibly tour New York City?

Out of our conversation, Franny came up with her answer – she was going to find a job in New York and make some money to calm her nerves. So on the day I had set to go to the surgical pathology department at Presbyterian Hospital, she was determined to go into the center of New York and find out if work was easy to find—or maybe just impossible as she knew absolutely nobody in the business world of New York.

Now here we were, July of 1946. Franny and I had just crossed over the George Washington Bridge and gotten into a subway. I got off at 168th Street and Franny stayed on, to go to downtown New York City and try to find a job. We planned to discuss our first day in New York City with each other when we got together later in the day at our room in Englewood, New Jersey, where we had found a place to live.

There was no problem finding the New York Presbyterian Hospital and no difficulty getting on an elevator and reaching the surgical pathology department on the 18th floor. Walking into the area where there was nothing but tables on which microscopes were set, many having young men or women looking through these machines at "something." I asked one young man if he could direct me to Dr. Stout's office and without hesitation he walked me a short distance and pointed. I promptly recognized Dr. Stout's office and introduced myself to his secretary.

Dr. Stout saw me immediately and proceeded to walk me back into the wide room which housed the tables, chairs, stools, young working people, and showed me one of those tables on which was a microscope covered with plastic of some kind, and behind it an empty stool. This area, I was then told, would be my "working" area; and Dr. Stout returned to his office.

What to do then? But that thought did not require a personal decision as a nice young man stepped over to me, introduced himself, and proceeded to tell me many things about the surgical pathology area, as he knew instantly that I was new to the area and could use a little help.

Things worked out just perfectly! Just what was I going to learn at the Presbyterian Hospital? What did I think that I should or could learn there? How did I think that going to the Columbia-Presbyterian Hospital in New York City was going to help me in the practice of surgery? And soon I had the answers to these several questions; and I never felt better having made the decision to accept the no-pay year in the surgical pathology department at Presbyterian New York City Hospital. My newly found friends in the surgical pathology division of the institution had obviously talked about having individuals already working there talk to and with me.

Individuals here would be offered a variety of microscopic slides to inspect via their microscopes, decide exactly what they had looked at, and keep proper but specific notes. They would have been initially informed about the surgical decision to operate and then asked to agree or not concerning what should or should not have been surgically performed. On many cases of infection or tumor problems, these individuals (I now one of them) would be asked as to how each of these cases could or should be managed: surgery, nothing, medical, radiation, re-biopsy – whatever. And then Dr. Stout would offer his personal opinion and be available to any one of us to question his decision, and remain available for any type of discussion.

Personally, I was extremely impressed by the fact that this famous Dr. Stout spent untold hours in this pathology room, obviously just teaching this group of whomevers – pathologists-to-be, medical personnel, or surgeons-to-be? But – there were many other things for this group of whomevers to do and learn about. And why would these individuals be spending so much time in a surgical pathology department? Good question. Some were hospital residents in the hospital and were paid a specific amount each month. Others, such as I, were in the surgical pathology area to learn to be good or better surgeons who could handle tumors or infectious problems better and were not being paid a cent. One other comment; the hospital residents, as just noted, were a portion of interns or residents, who were personally known and who had hospital cards that were used to pay for all their food, which they could pick up and eat right there. I was one of the few who had no "food card," but I got rather hungry at times. Since I had somewhat quickly gotten to know a few of those boys with food cards, and they didn't use them all the time, I discovered that they didn't mind loaning their cards to me rather frequently. I kept being lucky.

I have not said very much about what the individuals in Dr. Stout's great surgical pathology area were planning for later lives. Were some of these surgeons-to-be just planning so that they could make more money by learning much more about surgical pathology, or were they just going to be plain honest and hardworking surgeons? Time would tell.

After this day number one for me in my new position, five o'clock came and I was anxious to get back to our room in Englewood and very anxious to listen to what Franny had found out in New York about work for herself. This day continued to be not only an interesting day, it was just an unusual and super-interesting day – for both of us. I really wanted to find out whether or not Franny had gotten a job. The answer was that she had gotten a job, but not in downtown New York City.

The beginning of Franny's story was more than a little interesting but it just kept getting more than just interesting – it was unbelievable.

Franny had seen in the daily paper that secretaries were needed at one business – "please let us talk with you and see you." She chose to see and talk with those in that particular business in an extremely tall building – the Empire State Building. This discussion with her was long but good.

Franny chose to take an elevator to the office number that she had seen in the city newspaper. The beginning of a problem began when the elevator stopped on the 49th floor and quite clear information had her take the next door elevator to the top of that office building, the 60th floor. No time was lost in being seen by the man who was interviewing applicants, but he had no opportunity to ask Franny question number one. She instantly stated that she would like to thank him for seeing her so promptly, but that she had absolutely no interest in being a working girl there – the office was far too high. She right that minute was afraid she was going to be sick and she was going back down – one or two elevators to get down? "Thank you, but goodbye."

A big surprise, but minimal, compared to the discussion by Franny that followed. "Yes, I was scared to death and was never going to work in a big building, but I got a good job." Franny made that shocking statement: "I got a good job." I said, "Tell me about your job?"

And with that, I continued to be shocked, in a positive fashion. Her job was just more than perfect – hard to believe. Without waiting another minute, Franny gave me the nicest story.

"I came back to Presbyterian Hospital and found an area on the lobby floor where several ladies were sitting and I felt sure they were working for the hospital. I went over to them, introduced myself to them and asked them if they had any idea how I might find some kind of work. I briefly told them that my husband, you, was a new worker – not making any money in the lab up above – and that I needed a job.

"They could not have been nicer. They told me to go over to the Vanderbilt Clinic and see if they had anything to offer. After telling them that I didn't even know where the Vanderbilt Clinic was, they smiled and showed me which door to go through, as the Vanderbilt Clinic actually was part of the Presbyterian Hospital. And so, I went over to this Vanderbilt Clinic, found another desk behind which an older lady sat and asked her how I could get in touch with the office so that I could talk with those there about work.

"The talk in the office to which I was directed, was just plain good. I was sent to another area – I don't know anything about the area – but a nice man had me sit down and we talked. To make this story short, I got a job. And not just a job. I then became secretary to the director of the Vanderbilt Clinic. Can you believe this?" Mr. Thoms was my boss!

But – here we were – in a strange position. Completely new work for both of us, but we were completely happy that not only were we together after a very long time – World War II – but we now had positions in almost the same building, almost the same floor. Franny would right then be in a financial situation that would allow us to go out and get big hamburgers.

Back to my so-called work in the surgical pathology department and what I would be doing on a routine day. Each individual examined via his microscope numerous biopsy materials, often seeing the gross specimens. Teaching was via the senior resident among the group who would check with each individual and help with his or her education regarding surgical pathology in a variety of ways. We were asked to help as an assistant to surgeons on some occasions and on a regular basis, run the slide projector when Dr. Jerome Webster, professor of plastic surgery at Columbia Presbyterian, had his weekly meeting with his surgical residents. When it was my turn to show the slides, I was completely bored: how could any surgeon want to work at performing face-lifts, revising scars, and reducing the size of breasts? Little did I know that two years later, I would be in training in plastic surgery under the teaching of Dr. S. Milton Dupertuis. Dr. Dupertuis had been Dr. Webster's first plastic surgery resident at Columbia Presbyterian and some years later, Dr. Webster and I became quite good friends – he often referred to me as his grandson. Many years later, we even played golf together – the last time was in Australia. Often the past situations have to be difficult even to believe.

Much more about plastic surgery soon and that will involve plastic surgery and money.

Mentioning names means telling stories. One of the best things I ever learned about medicine and surgery and complete honesty is related at this moment. The chief resident in the department of orthopedic surgery was Dr. Bill Lehman, a superior young individual in almost anything one could place him – but I put him number one as being just honest, sincere, and a superior teacher. He and I in some way respected the fashion in which we approached and loved every aspect of the teaching and learning of surgical pathology. We became friends for this very reason. We loved what we worked in and for – pathology. And almost to the minute, we knew that the two of us would do some type of surgical pathology together somewhat promptly – and we did. Both of us were interested in one very important pathology item. There were untold numbers of tuberculosis and Boeck's sarcoid microscopic slides available describing those specific diseases. But relatively recently, as of that date, medical articles were beginning to appear that were somewhat disturbing: the diagnosis of tuberculosis in many instances was wrong. The correct diagnosis was Boeck's sarcoid, which made doctors reflect upon all the money spent to take care of tubercular cases when there was no specific treatment for Boeck's sarcoid. (Of course, Bill and I knew that we were right, and all those who thought otherwise obviously were wrong.)

Bill and I spent many Saturday afternoons microscopically comparing all the slides of tuberculosis and Boeck's sarcoid, which slides had resided there at Presbyterian Hospital for years. It was at that particular time that it was then technically possible to tell the difference between those two diseases microscopically, and it was clear that many, too many, cases of tuberculosis were diagnosed that actually were Boeck's sarcoid. After several months, extremely pleased with ourselves, we took our completed work to Dr. Stout, expecting a pat on the back. Dr. Stout asked us what we thought that we had accomplished, and we told him, that we had proven absolutely that we had more cases of Boeck's sarcoid than any published work.

Dr. Stout then asked us how this knowledge, more proven cases of Boeck's sarcoid than any other author, would benefit people. We, of course, had to answer that it would not help people, but that we could say Presbyterian Hospital had the most cases, to which Dr Stout quietly said, "Your work is good, but we won't publish it; that would just clutter up the literature." This was a real disappointment after months of hard work, but a lesson we would never forget. (In 2009, I still could never forget this.)

Every day was not like every other day. This particular day, my group of young men and women – and I of course was one of the young men – had something to do that would specifically involve Dr. Stout. I don't have any idea who dreamed this up but the plan was quite interesting. As noted earlier, each and every one who was in the "workroom" of this surgical pathology area looked up to Dr. Stout and would never do anything but show this to him.

What we had done was to take a hot dog, cut it exactly the way a tumor was cut, and place it on a glass slide to make it look like the type of microscopic slides that were being examined during many hours of the day. Dr. Stout was then called and asked to come into this workroom. One of this group of smart young individuals was chosen to present this slide to Dr. Stout, which he did, saying that after many of us had examined this slide, we could not diagnose what was thought to be a tumor. We really wanted the opinion of Dr. Stout, really thinking that he would come up with the name of some kind of a fancy, unique tumor.

Dr. Stout took the slide, sat down behind a microscope, slid his glasses off, and studied this slide in his usual professional fashion. After some minutes, he sat back on his stool, gently pushed the microscope away, placed his glasses back on, and said quietly but in an absolutely professional voice, "I know that this is a hot dog, but I'm just not sure if it comes from the Chicago stockyards." And with that, Dr. Stout rose from his stool, thanked us for asking for his opinion regarding the slide, and quietly walked over to his private office.

This visit by Dr. Stout was the first and last time this young group ever tried to stick Dr. Stout in any fashion: We all just thought much more of our superior boss. It was just quite obvious to all of us that our Dr. Arthur Purdy Stout was not only a superior medical physician but also a superior gentleman.

But everything was not just hard work every day – or maybe hard work was on the way. One day, I had been assigned to work on the 19th floor, just above our area on the 18th floor. Our work, if called work and not just research, was usually just routine, but this particular day it wasn't just routine. I went down the hall on the 18th floor, to the room that housed live material for research purposes. I took a small monkey out of an area, put him casually under my arm, and returned to our lab to get something when suddenly this little monkey jumped away from my arm, sprang up on the table and jumped out of an open window. What to do? I did it without delay.

I grabbed a bag of some kind, so that I could pick up the remains of this monkey after I had taken the elevator down 18 floors, went outside to pick up the various parts of the monkey who had fallen 18 floors and landed on solid cement. To my absolute surprise, this dumb monkey was just sitting there, arms waving, apparently just waiting to be picked up. So, I picked him up, stuck him under my arm again – he was not injured in any obvious way – and took an elevator back to the 18th floor. Animal surgery was postponed for me that day.

I promptly learned something about monkeys. They are put together much differently than humans and most other animals that live among trees. The hand-like portion is attached to the mid body by a wide band of skin that can and does function like a parachute, so this little monkey had just spread his legs when he jumped out of that window on the 18th floor at the Presbyterian Hospital in New York City and floated to safety. I just seemed to learn more and more every day.

My tasks were many and varied, but always interesting and instructive. Initially, as noted earlier, I disliked having been chosen to show the slides for the plastic surgery residents on Friday afternoons – such a non-important specialty. In addition, Franny had to take dictation, from the same plastic surgery residents; they had to do their dictation in the Vanderbilt Clinic, when they elected to transfer patients they preferred not to treat to the free city hospitals (Bellevue, Mauresania, etc.). These plastic surgery residents eventually were chosen, because of superior ability, to guide the specialty of plastic surgery in the entire country. Some of these men were Drs. Bill Littler, Sammy Paletta, Art Aufsis, Bill Whelan and others – still some of the best-known surgeons in the world – and we all became good friends years later.

We made friends among the resident and hospital staffs at Presbyterian, one resident in particular being Ken Hui, a Chinese boy from Hong Kong. Later that year, he became the chief resident in general surgery at Presbyterian. Ken was extremely easy to get to know and we began to see him for visits. He was not married then and began to take us out for dinner, once or twice a week. Ken knew the owners and kitchen staffs of some excellent Chinese restaurants and it was to these restaurants where he took us – we ate free in all of these expensive type kitchens. More about Ken later, when he became chairman of the department of surgery at the Queen of Angels Hospital in Hong Kong.

On that New Year's Eve, Franny and I had a big night. We took the subway downtown to Times Square to watch that big "something" being dropped down at midnight. Never to be forgotten! We never considered being alone in this place or the other during that period of time. We actually walked alone, at night, in any part of New York City and felt comfortable. A good walk was one down 125th Street to Harlem.

I saw Dr. Pool regularly. He would come up to Presbyterian Hospital every couple of weeks and we would eat lunch. One night, Franny and I had dinner with the Pools at their home on 76th Street. John was called and he agreed to make a house call – at the Waldorf Towers Hotel. The patient? Henry Fonda! John had reverted to the practice of lung surgery upon his return to New York City.

After leaving New York City in June of 1947, I continued to keep in touch with John Pool. We had enjoyed a close friendship that began when fate brought us together in a field hospital. It is a friendship that has lasted sixty years. I owe so much to him, in so many ways. He shaped my surgical life in countless ways, and I will always hold him in high esteem. He is truly a great man.

8 || RESIDENT – GENERAL SURGERY – PITTSBURGH

I was one of the fortunate ones who made it back to the United States after a terrible war. I look back with only one regret: I wish that I had been able to save more lives.

June of 1947 found me in Pittsburgh as a resident in general surgery. Teaching was not productive but it turned out to be a good year for me in a variety of ways.

Lots of good weather in June of 1947 and were there not some golf courses? And hadn't I played a little golf a few years ago?

> **GOLF AND MEDICINE**
>
> It is a science – the study of a lifetime, in which you may exhaust yourself but never your subject.
>
> It is a contest, a duel or a melee, calling for courage, skill, strategy and self-control.
>
> It is a test of temper, a trial of honor, a revealer of character.
>
> It affords a chance to play the man and act the gentleman.
>
> It means going into God's out-of-doors, getting close to nature, fresh air, exercise, a sweeping away of the mental cobwebs, genuine recreation of the tired tissues.
>
> It is a cure for care – an antidote to worry.
>
> It includes companionship with friends, social intercourse, opportunity for courtesy, kindliness and generosity to an opponent.
>
> It promotes not only physical health, but moral force.
>
> David R. Forgan (circa 1930)

THE PRACTICE OF MEDICINE

Work and learning certainly are not over after graduating from medical school and completing the required minimum hospital experience. Work and learning are absolutely continuous. The rules are there to be followed. Modern textbooks and never-ending journals are available to be read. To keep up to date on a chosen specialty, regular attendance at professional meetings to listen to the leaders is unquestionably mandatory.

Four months of that year for me were on the gynecology service in the Women's Hospital, now part of Presbyterian. The men for whom and with whom I worked were an unusually good group. They were well aware of the fact that general surgery, not gynecological surgery, was my goal, so that they were not adverse to permitting me to admit general surgical cases (gallbladders, thyroids, parotids, and almost any type of general surgery) to their services. While they did not scrub in the operating room with me, presumably they would have been held responsible for any surgical problems should they have occurred.

The one bright spot in this year of general surgery was the friendship I developed with the chairman of the department of surgery, Dr. Sam Harbison. While Dr. Harbison (and it quickly became Sam, not Professor Harbison) did very little surgery himself, he made a valiant effort to develop a surgical training program, but it was a failed effort. I recall that Sam managed to have the hospital buy an air conditioning unit for his operating room in Presbyterian – the first time an operating room at Women's or Presbyterian Hospital was cooled. That meant that there was no need in that room for an extra nurse to mop sweaty brows and the surgeon did not have to roll up his pants in an effort to keep his temperature under control. It must seem unimaginable for a surgeon in 2009 that in 1947 operating rooms were like ovens.

Sam and I played an occasional game of golf together, and one day I told him about my long time interest in head and neck surgery. He was informed about the fact that Dr. Hays Martin, without question the father of head and neck surgery, had offered me the head and neck surgical residency at Memorial Hospital in New York City and that I had not accepted it, electing to be in Pittsburgh. Following this discussion, Sam suggested that I work out some kind of program with Dr. Martin in New York so that I could really learn head and neck surgery.

There was no difficulty arranging work at Memorial. I would take the train at night to New York with a fare of about $6.00 one way, reach Pennsylvania Station about 7:00 AM and go straight to Memorial. I would attend the clinics, watch and work in the operating rooms, borrow meal tickets, find an empty bed, and would love every minute of it. This was one of the greatest experiences of my surgical life and would be the basis for my surgery the remainder of my career.

The so-called general surgery residency program at the University of Pittsburgh in 1947 was really not a training program. There was no organized teaching, but the young surgeon cannot depend on others to hand feed him. Certainly help and teaching should be provided, but the one learning must teach himself to teach himself, and there will always be ways to do this.

An article in the *Pittsburgh Tribune Review* daily paper of May 31, 1999 caught my eye. Katie Couric, host of NBC's "Today Show," speaking at commencement at Lehigh University on May 30 said "— work should feel like play, because getting that brass ring is no fun if you don't enjoy the merry-go-round."

Don't be afraid to expend a little more effort and become better. It isn't necessary to have everything handed to you. Why not make things happen?

Sometimes odd but interesting things do happen. After my several months at Women's Hospital, I only had to walk around the corner from those operating rooms and I was in Presbyterian Hospital – and each hospital, one big building, had its own board of directors.

And several "odd" things did happen. The chief resident in general surgery at Presbyterian Hospital, at this time, was a nice guy and a good surgeon, but he had another job. His name was Danny Fortman, captain of the famous Chicago Bears professional football team. That meant that there were a number of weekends in the fall when Danny had to turn the necessary surgical problems over to another surgical resident, usually me–as you know where he was spending his weekends.

By the time seven or eight months had passed, I was quite certain that when I had finished my general surgery residency I would be out in practice attempting to develop a practice in surgery, chiefly head and neck but also pediatric surgery.

But strange things can happen to young surgeons and I was no exception in my general surgery residency.

Dr. S. Milton Dupertuis, chief of plastic surgery, had an operation scheduled and no assistant to help him. Plastic surgery was not an important specialty in Pittsburgh; there was no training program, and Dr. Dupertuis did not rate a surgical resident helper. However, part of my job as a senior resident in general surgery was to assign interns and residents as assistants to practicing general surgeons. But, because Dr. Dupertuis' operation was an extremely extensive and potentially dangerous one (reconstruction of a cervical esophagus), I offered to scrub with him. The surgical procedure went extremely smoothly, and I was impressed by the technical ability of Dr. Dupertuis and the thought behind this complicated operation. The patient was a young woman from Europe who, for some unknown reason, had drunk some material similar to American Clorox (sodium hypochlorite, sodium hydroxide, sodium silicate, etc.). As a result, this had prevented her from swallowing anything, including her saliva and had necessitated a gastrostomy (a feeding tube having been inserted into her stomach from outside her body.)

A number of days went by and I continued to go over the technical points of the operation recently performed by Dr. Dupertuis. When Dr. Dupertuis was asked if I might assist him on a few additional operative procedures, the answer was a rather quick "yes." Within a very brief interval my mind was made up regarding a specialty I had labeled, as a fellow in pathology in New York, as rather unimportant and really stupid. I approached Dr. Dupertuis one day with the question as to whether he had ever considered attempting to develop a residency training program in plastic and reconstructive surgery. He answered by saying that he had not given that idea much thought because he really didn't think there would be much interest in such a program. My answer to that was that there was a sincere interest in the planning of such a residency, and if he would accept me as his first plastic surgery resident, I would help him build the service. He made an immediate decision to proceed with an attempt to gain prompt approval for such a training program and as of that moment, plans began to be formulated. How lucky could a young, naïve surgical resident be? But, a quote by William Arthur Ward is worth requoting: "Opportunities are like sunrises. If you wait too long, you miss them."

Dr. Dupertuis stated that he had just completed arrangements for a Philadelphia surgeon to join him as an assistant but that those plans would not militate against a residency program start-up. The name of the assistant-to-be was Dr. Willie White. At this particular time in the United States there were but very few residency positions in the entire country. Now there are hundreds of plastic surgery residents scattered in American training programs. Most practicing plastic surgeons as of that era had assistants working with them.

It was obvious that the three of us could work together. It was also quite clear that Dr. Dupertuis was going to be adopting a personal surgical program of cosmetic type procedures while Dr. White and I were on the other side of the fence in this specialty. We would work on the reconstructive side. Almost immediately we made known our surgical preferences and Dr. Dupertuis was delighted. This genuine discussion from that moment was the best thing that could have developed. From that day, Dr. White's name became "Willie," not William or Doctor.

The plastic surgery residency, as outlined by the American Board of Plastic Surgery, was two years in length, and the rules and regulations that outlined what a resident should learn to do in those two years were clearly presented. The first statement was that the resident had to have had a general internship following graduation from medical school, followed by five years of residency training in general surgery. In addition, before the trained plastic surgery resident could take the qualifying American Board of Plastic Surgery examination, he had to have practiced plastic surgery for two years, and he had to have taken and passed the American Board of General Surgery.

The plastic surgery training program was exactly what I wanted, even though I had no pre-conceived plans. Willie and I worked together with no problems. We would study surgical books and began performing operations that were not really being carried out in Pittsburgh in any acceptable or superior fashion. One day Willie said, "Let's do the surgery that no one is doing in Pittsburgh." He was referring to hand surgery and head and neck surgery. Willie was correct. There was not one hand surgeon and but one surgeon carrying out any head and neck surgery in Pittsburgh or any surrounding areas. This prompted Willie to say, "Which type of surgeon do you want to be?" And my answer was "head and neck." From that day on we began plans to become absolutely the best surgeons in those two areas of study.

Falk Clinic of the University of Pittsburgh was a prime source of patient material. There were untold numbers of clinic patients with hand problems such as unrepaired severed tendons, tumors, and congenital deformities, which problems had gone untreated or been managed in less than acceptable ways for countless years. The head and neck situation was similar. These cases were parotid tumors, cancer of the tongue, larynx, upper and lower jaws and many other problems. X-ray therapy, instead of surgery, had been used to treat many non-cancerous diseases or tumors resulting in a huge number of radio-necrotic (dead) bones, particularly facial bones. The sheer number of people to be operated on was overpowering, but Willie and I, with Dr. Dupertuis's backing, knew what could and should be done.

Willie had previously spent some time with one of the world's most famous hand surgeons, Dr. Sterling Bunnell of California, so that he had an excellent background in hands. My exposure to head and neck problems was not extensive, but things changed immediately. So that my knowledge of hand surgery would be acceptable, it was arranged for me to spend a number of weeks at Passavant Hospital in Chicago on the hand service. That experience was phenomenal, as my teachers there were Drs. Koch, Mason and Allen – three fine gentlemen, surgeons and instructors. I lived at the YMCA but was paid by the Presbyterian Hospital of Pittsburgh. As chief resident in plastic surgery there I was paid $100 a month, but no more free food or a bed at Presbyterian when I was in Pittsburgh. After the Chicago hiatus, I continued to commute to New York to absorb as much knowledge as possible at New York Memorial Hospital on every variety of head and neck tumors, the most important and interesting period of my medical life. (How could I possibly think that in 1978, I would become President of the Society of Head and Neck Surgeons?)

The residency program became stronger each year. Applicants were numerous and we had the good fortune of being placed in the position that we could pick and choose from among them. And we made some excellent choices.

Although I was among the so-called "teachers" in the plastic surgery residency program, as the years went by, it became quite apparent that most of our residents did not learn all their good points from us. A number of our fine young new plastic surgeons eventually became quite important medically. To me, nothing could be more rewarding than to watch a former surgical resident develop and pass his teachers in various aspects of his specialty.

And again, why did I believe a resident should be assigned to Dr. Dupertuis for assistance in a cervical esophagus reconstruction operation? Possibly because as chief resident in pediatric surgery at Pittsburgh Children's Hospital in 1943, I had by the Grace of God, successfully performed an identical procedure on a little boy, and Dr. Dupertuis needed all the help possible. Such experiences are never forgotten.

And why did the plastic surgery training program begin in 1948 and not 1945 or 1960? It was just by sheer accident, as earlier described. And this training program was quite different from other types of surgical training programs in Pittsburgh. Pittsburgh, during the 1940s and 1950s, was woefully behind the times in any type of surgical training, particularly general surgery. In 1942, there were no general surgery residents at the University of Pittsburgh Presbyterian and Women's Hospitals and one medical resident.

9 || SURGERY & MONEY

It is my personal opinion that Dr. S. Milton Dupertuis was the one man responsible for what was considered to be an exceptional plastic surgery training program. He was looked up to by his peers as a gentleman, completely honest, and a hard-working superior surgeon. Residents trained by Milt Dupertuis were most fortunate to have had him as a mentor.

In 1951, I became certified by the American Board of General Surgery. That made it possible to take the qualifying Board in Plastic and Reconstructive Surgery, which I took and passed in New York City in 1952. It is of interest at this time to realize that in 1952, there were but eleven candidates who took that examination, while in 2006, several hundred took it. This would make one think that plastic surgery was a very new type of surgery in the 40s and 50s, but in reality it was the oldest.

It is actually quite difficult for me to believe what has happened regarding the specialty of so-called plastic surgery—just the fact that there are hundreds of plastic surgeons in the United States today when in the 1940s there were just a handful. I was one of this "handful" of trained plastic surgeons (a total of 12) taking the oral examination in New York City in 1952.

At this time, I would like to discuss the specialty of plastic surgery on a personal level. Golf and business will be included in this so-called presentation, as I believe my background as a member of the American Board of Plastic Surgery, from May 1968 trough May 1974 and as vice chairman of the Board from June 1973 through May 1974, entitles me to a personal opinion.

Almost every individual believes that plastic surgery means cosmetic. Following are several descriptions of the words cosmetic, plastic, and plastic surgery. A Greek word, plastikos, is described also.

Cosmetic

a) serving to modify or improve the appearance of a physical feature, defect, or irregularity: cosmetic surgery

b) serving to beautify the body, especially the face and hair

Plastic – relating to or dealing with shaping or modeling

Plastic Surgery – surgery to remodel, repair, or restore body parts, especially by the transfer of tissue

Plastikos (Greek) – forming, growing, changing, developing

Plastic surgery for many years was considered to be the oldest specialty in surgery in the world. Various descriptions of the word plastic in a number of books means return to normal. The specialty of plastic surgery for years was known as the type of surgery that would return the individual to a normal state, should he not be in an acceptable normal state as the result of birth defects, infections, or accidents. Unfortunately, plastic surgery today often means cosmetic surgery.

The change in the meaning of the words plastic surgery has radically changed the type of surgery that plastic surgeons performed in the relatively recent past. The name of plastic and reconstructive surgery is now gone and the type of surgery that has been performed for many years is actually a thing of the past. The vast majority of plastic surgeons are not in any way interested in or even capable of performing acceptable surgery for numerous physical situations. A few of the medical problems these new type plastic surgeons have no interest in or ability to manage surgically are: 1) congenital problems, 2) traumatic problems such as fractures and soft tissue trauma, 3) tumors of the head and neck, 4) soft tissue tumors, and a list of other situations.

There is one major reason why the majority (vast majority) of plastic surgeons – and they are not known as plastic and reconstructive surgeons – do not perform the surgery just described in the preceding and current chapters. These plastic surgeons are only interested in making money.

Money means many reasons as to why doctors do a variety of things. This does not always happen in the United States of America. Money brings things to people! But how far away could a money situation really happen, and how could it be truly connected with medicine – and is this specifically related to plastic surgery? Money is a very important part of the medical practice of many doctors in every specialty.

Anyone even remotely connected with hospitals, operating rooms, training programs and patient care in particular must be acutely aware of how the practice of medicine has changed over the past twenty years. There is no question that the medical profession has lost its elevated position in the eyes of the general public, even though people are living longer, healthier lives because of the care they have received from many great physicians. Then what are the problems? This is what I hoped to find out in various interviews.

My respect for doctors is enormous, yet I do not agree with a lot of decisions they make regarding non-medical business and I delight in never-ending discussions with them on a wide variety of subjects. Doctors relish always being correct, whether it be a ruling in golf, the better car to drive – Ford or Lincoln—or why the hospital administration made such a dumb decision about some new piece of equipment. Some discussions remind me of the song by Mac Davis, "It's Hard to be Humble When You're Perfect in Every Way." Physicians are a breed of their own. Obviously, there are exceptions to the rule, but generally speaking, the average doctor is prone to argue; he has a somewhat inflated opinion of himself; and he is not a good listener.

The classic book *How to Win Friends and Influence People* by Dale Carnegie has a lot to say about being a good listener. Carnegie says that if you aspire to be a good conversationalist, you must first be an attentive listener. Henry Ford attributed personal success to being a good listener: "If there is any one secret of success, it lies in the ability to get the other person's point of view and see things from that person's angle as well as your own."

In February of 1972, much was learned regarding money at Witwattersrand University in Johannesburg, South Africa. That superior university invited me to spend some time there with a group of surgeons, with the vast amount of time discussing head and neck tumor problems. I possibly learned more about surgeons in South Africa than the medical individuals learned from me.

I asked if these university surgeons taught their surgical residents everything they could regarding head and neck tumors. Many of their surgical residents lived in a variety of areas, and had no relationship with the city of Johannesburg. I was told that close to 100 percent of these surgeons, who were trained in cancer surgery, never returned to the university so that they could remain up-to-date with the specialty. They were just interested in one thing – money. And here it was – money – the identical problem that involved so many surgeons in the United States.

This subject, money, appears to remain a very popular subject. A really interesting subject just came to mind. In 1964, a small group of plastic surgeons and one non-medical man met one evening in Houston, Texas. This group included Dr. Tom Cronin of Houston, now deceased, Dr. Robert MacCormick, professor of surgery at the University of Rochester, Dr. Tom Reese, professor of surgery at New York University, Dr. Milton Edgerton, professor of surgery at Johns Hopkins University, Mr. Silas Braley, a representative of Dow Corning Corporation and me. (Silas Braley was actually from Pittsburgh and over a number of months, he and I became good friends, as I was later working on tendon grafts, and the words "silastic rods" came up. The company Silas worked for, Dow Corning, made silastic material and named it "silastic" in honor of Silas Braley.) The purpose of this meeting was to discuss whether or not it might be reasonable to use silicone prosthesis to enlarge or reconstruct the female breast. Silicone was a Dow Corning product. The decision that night was that Cronin, Edgerton and Reese would operate on a few chosen candidates and then we would meet and discuss the results. A number of cases were completed, but the initial plan was not followed.

Word quickly got around about this silicone procedure and Dow Corning immediately supplied the requested implants. There was never a second meeting of this group. Many years later, the question arose as to why basic clinical research was not carried out to determine the safety of implanting silicone foreign bodies. The answer is quite clear. While the FDA (Food and Drug Administration) currently determines the right to use new surgical products, called devices, the FDA did not have this authoritative control until March of 1984.

It is well known that countless lawsuits followed as a result of the implanting of silicone material. That has been going on for years. My cosmetic surgery interests never involved breast augmentative techniques so that my problems with this material were nil.

Hundreds upon hundreds of medico-legal situations resulted as the techniques of silicone implants into female breasts progressed, and this problem was still a problem in various ways in 2008, somewhat less in 2009.

Physicians are generally held in high regard, mainly because people assume that physicians exist to help those in need. Of course, there are always exceptions, and a fascinating book called *The Doctors* addresses the negative aspects of the medical profession. Published in 1962 and unfortunately now out of print, the book is surprisingly current in many of its observations and is a powerful wake-up call to all students of medicine, doctors in training, and those in practice or in research. The *Los Angeles Herald Examiner* called the book, "a provocative sizzler written by a researcher who likes to slip time bombs under sacred covers."

The Doctors makes some astonishing claims, "shattering revelations that show why the American physician is scientifically, intellectually, and humanly ill-equipped for modern medical practice."

The author of *The Doctors*, Mr. Martin L. Gross, wrote in a most provocative manner. Many of his comments were extremely stated, but most probably could fit numerous doctors.

Mr. Gross was quite specific, saying that doctors had an income four times that of the average family. Some doctors would agree with Mr. Gross. When I interviewed one resident, he had this to say: "I want to do some kind of procedural work. There are all types of technical things to do in radiology and surgery, lots of real fancy work. And money is definitely a factor. The way it looks now I'm going to have about $200,000 in loans to pay back after graduation form Temple, that alone makes me want to be in a specialty part of medicine and make more money."

I was surprised to learn that this bright young man knew absolutely nothing about medical laws. He had not been involved in any discussions at medical school, or at West Penn Hospital.

We talked about the Burn/Trauma Center and why there were so few medical doctors on staff, and why there were so few burn centers in general. I told him that burn centers had always been considered money losers by the hospitals and that the vast majority of doctors wanted nothing to do with handling burn victims. Very few hospital personnel or physicians had any desire to become involved with burn patients. There were several real reasons for this lack of interest. For countless years, no training was offered in how to adequately manage the burn patient. The burn victim usually had limited financial resources and minimal insurance for a long-term hospital stay and the medical care itself was costly and time-consuming.

Mr. Gross went on and on about the many things that physicians did which were just improper. These things, just to briefly mention a few, were that doctors experiment on humans without their consent, train at second class medical schools, make lots of money and live a life far above the average citizens.

Of course, everyone knows that there are no medical problems today and that everyone loves and respects his personal physician, enjoys his hospital stays, and has absolutely no complaints. Everything is just fine, right? Dream on!

I share some of the quotes from *The Doctors* because of their relevance today and because of their usefulness in forcing all of us in the medical profession to do some serious soul-searching. It must be recognized, however, that the book presents every possible unacceptable situation faced by patients and physicians. Still, many of those situations may be all too familiar to us today.

Many books have been written by outstanding doctors that attest to the honesty and nobility of the medical profession. Certainly they far outnumber books like The Doctors that present the opposing view. There are plenty of medical individuals who earn millions throughout their career, but most of them have earned every dollar they have ever received. The fact that a physician has a huge bank account should in no way lead one to assume that the physician has performed in a spurious or otherwise unacceptable fashion. Perhaps the bank account grew because the physician discovered a profitable medical technique, inherited money from a wealthy relative, invested well, or was just plain lucky.

It was Dale Carnegie's encouragement to talk about "one's own mistakes" that prompted me to describe a variety of my own experiences, which discussions extended over several sessions.

There is a weekly meeting at the West Penn Hospital Burn/Trauma Center, where a speaker presents a variety of topics. The so-called audience may include medical students, interns, residents, nurses, or anyone who has some connection with or is interested in burn unit situations. I talked at this morning meeting a number of times. Following are some of my Saturday morning talks. I had told a number of the interns and residents that I was going to present some of my surgical work on a couple of Saturdays so I'm certain they all thought that I would present some great cases. Do you think that they may have been surprised, a little, when these cases were presented? Some of the surgical work performed by me and discussion that followed are outlined.

CASE 1

When a newborn baby was admitted to the hospital with a rather large section of brain exposed, I was not aware that it was then the considered opinion that death would occur promptly from brain hemorrhage if the brain was not covered by the patient's own skin. Fortunately, a medical resident had read about this and informed me. I promptly placed a large skin graft over the brain and the baby survived.

If that medical resident had not told me about that brain problem, that newborn baby would have died.

CASE 2

One doesn't have to be a beginner to get into problems. In 1944, when I served as assistant chief of surgery of the 92nd Field Hospital in the Philippines, a young boy was brought in bleeding, having been shot in the chest. No problem – just a damaged interstitial artery. No problem until I found that the boy was going downhill fast and bleeding from a damaged right lower lung.

In surgery, prompt decisions are often necessary. This was one of those times. Two ribs were divided, the wound spread very wide, and the lower part of the right lower lobe was removed. This boy had all of this done under local anesthesia, and he was more dead than alive at that time.

This was the only lung that I have ever operated on, but we both survived.

Had I been a little smarter, it would have been apparent that this situation was not a simple one but very serious, and I would have had time to awaken the chief surgeon of the 92nd, Dr. John Pool, a well-known New York city chest surgeon who would have placed the patient at far less risk.

CASE 3

As I was in the surgical department at West Penn, a doctor in a nearby town referred a patient to me who had cancer of the tongue. The man had a definite, large non-ulcerated tumor on the tongue. He had had this tumor biopsied and showed me the pathologist's typed report, which identified the tumor as "squamous cell cancer."

I performed a partial glossectomy on the man. The pathology report came back "granular cell myoblastoma," a tumor that is *not* malignant.

And why am I telling you this story? First, if you are going to be performing head and neck tumor surgery, or even other types of tumor work, you *better* become well versed in surgical pathology right away... this is mandatory!

Secondly, I made a grave error in not requesting that the microscopic slides from the original biopsy be sent to my surgical pathology department at West Penn Hospital for the opinion of those who were expert in head and neck tumor pathology.

As for this particular case, the surgery that was undertaken was proper for a non-malignant tongue tumor. The patient and I were both lucky that the end result of my treatment did good and not harm.

CASE 4

When I was a general surgery resident at Pittsburgh Women's Hospital in the 1940s, we were offered short periods of training in gynecology. One evening, I was called to see a young woman who seemed to be in the throes of an incomplete abortion. However, the patient was adamant – "never been pregnant!" I tugged on the presenting part of the fetus but couldn't get it out.

I placed a call to the gynecologist, who suggested that I made sure the examining light was sufficiently bright. Check carefully and call back, the gynecologist said.

I did what I was told to do and then "called back" to report that the young lady was right. She was not pregnant; she had a prolapsed uterus, and of course, I couldn't pull it out.

CASE 5

There will never be perfect hospitals and doctors, but there are numerous good, smart doctors and great hospitals. This next medical problem involved a twenty-five-year-old girl who had had her right eye removed at Eye and Ear Hospital in Pittsburgh for a slowly progressive tumor-like growth and was beginning to develop a similar condition in the left eye. She was referred to me for an opinion and asked if I would consider removing her left eye.

The surgical pathology report from Eye and Ear Hospital shed no light on the nature of the tissue problem, failing to confirm a tumor or any pathology, and I was not prepared to perform any additional surgery. In order to avoid serious error, I thought it would be a good idea to get the opinion of a close friend, a plastic surgeon and head and necker, Dr. Milton Edgerton, chief of the Department of Plastic Surgery at Johns Hopkins University in Baltimore. The patient agreed to go to Johns Hopkins and was seen by Dr. Edgerton. Dr. Edgerton had no idea what was going on with this second eye but asked the senior resident in Ear, Nose and Throat Surgery there to look at the girl.

The Eye and Ear resident transferred this girl to a private room where an outsider could watch what was going on inside the room from a peephole.

And what did the resident see? This girl was purposely trying to destroy her remaining eye. We learned later that she was responsible for the loss of her right eye. Why? Who knows what goes on in the minds of seemingly "normal" people! But her case is not rare. In this case, Dr. Edgerton recommended psychiatric help, and the girl returned to Pittsburgh.

CASE 6

A young black male patient about thirty years old had a huge bedsore on his left hip. The skin there was black and dead looking. The man was a paraplegic and therefore had no sensation. He had been on the ward for quite some time and had obviously had extremely poor nursing care. We rotated an adjacent skin flap and did a free graft to replace the flap. The reconstruction was perfect.

Some time later, the man developed a bedsore in the area of the graft. The cause? More poor nursing care.

Who was responsible for this unacceptable result? The nurses, certainly, but I also blame myself for thinking that I had the problem permanently solved. I should have continued to visit that patient and I should have forced the issue of better nursing care.

CASE 7

It is generally known that surgeons mark the areas targeted for surgery, using material that is not easily erased so that incorrect surgical operations are not performed.

I recall an experience that was a near disaster. The patient was a young woman who had one very large breast and one that I thought perfectly suited her size and shape. On the way in to the operating room, I mentioned to the patient that the reduction in the size of that large breast would probably make her more comfortable. While her preoperative sedation was being dispensed, she told me in a loud voice that she wanted the smaller breast made larger, to match the big breast.

Surgery was canceled. The patient went home and eventually found another doctor.

CASE 8

About 1955, while I was on the surgical staff of the Veterans Hospital in Aspinwall, Pennsylvania, there was a man on the operating table; about to be operated on for a cancer about the size of a large orange that protruded several inches above the skin. Just as I was about to operate in the adjacent room, I happened to peer in at the protruding abdominal tumor next door. I commented that it would be impossible to remove such a cancer, but if they were to resect the abdominal wall, I could reconstruct it.

Somewhat later that morning, the surgeon operating on that tumor poked his head into my operating room. He had just finished the complete removal of the cancer, and as he took off his gloves, he said, "He's yours." Many times, it really pays to keep your mouth shut. Can't remember the reconstruction surgery it took to fix this abdomen.

CASE 9

One night while I was on call as a general surgery resident at the University of Pittsburgh Presbyterian Hospital, a forty-year-old man was admitted, having been transferred from a mental institution. I notified the surgeon on call that the patient was suffering from an obvious acute appendix. The man was scheduled for surgery at 10:00 PM and the senior surgeon arrived to assist me in performing the appendectomy.

Upon opening the abdomen, we discovered that a length of metal coat hanger had been inserted into the patient's abdomen via the anus.

Had I performed a rectal examination on this patient, I would have realized that he did not have appendicitis. But I didn't do that. The senior surgeon did not have anything to say to me about my unacceptable work – he knew that I had learned a lot.

CASE 10

In 1960, a well-dressed gentleman, age 55, sat down in my office across the desk from me. He was most polite as he pulled out a checkbook and fountain pen from his pocket, placed them on my desk, and said, "I'll pay you any amount of money if you will put scars on my face."

This was the first and only time a patient of mine ever made such an unusual request.

When I asked this person why he was requesting such an operation, he answered bluntly that he had a high position in one of Pittsburgh's big steel companies, was in line to go higher, but thought that if he had some facial scars, he would look stronger and would be in a better position to get that promotion.

I promptly told this man that it was my policy to refer individuals with unusual surgery requests to a psychiatrist before I would discuss surgery with them. The man accepted my approach and I made an appointment for him.

I just plain forgot about this until one day, a full year later, he returned to my office. This time, the patient did not pull out his checkbook. He sat across from me, smiling and obviously comfortable, and brought me up to date on his past year. He had seen the psychiatrist to whom I referred him, and had spent several sessions with him before returning to see me.

"I have done very well during the past year. The psychiatrist was superior. And I want to thank you for your approach to my initial request for facial scars. My steel mill job is just fine. Incidentally, I did not get promoted to that top job. Thank you!"

The Saturday morning groups all were more than a little surprised – some shocked – after reviewing these somewhat unusual cases. They had no idea that so many questionable situations had occurred as a result of the work by one who was there to teach. Several came to me and said they had learned a lot to hear their so-called teacher show his rather bad medical and surgical results.

The last few pages made it quite clear that I am one of more than just a few medical doctors who have made medical/surgical mistakes. The May 26, 2008 *American Medical News Journal* published a rather interesting study on the fact that only 9% of doctors practice in rural areas, while 20% of the population live there. And why do 90% of doctors elect to practice away from rural areas? — *money!*

My answer to the above article regarding rural doctors– Train those country doctors properly regarding proper patient care and have them be more interested in that patient care and less interested in money.

There is no question about "rural" doctors being sent to small towns and rural areas for training purposes. Many are planning to return from the country work and do a better job of medical care for city people. The real reason to leave a rural job and return to the city type medical practice? To make more money and to do less hard work.

This last article about having more medical doctors setting up their practices in the country or small towns, made me want to talk more about the training of resident doctors and doctors following their training. An article appeared in *JAMA* (*Journal of American Medical Association*), December 12, 2007 edition that was written by Arnold S. Relman, MD. This article was a true education, which caused me to agree completely with most of what Dr. Relman wrote.

Some of Dr Relman's statements are as follows:

> "...physicians accepted the view that medical practice is a business."

> "...the practice of medicine could only be conducted properly as a profession."

The description of a profession, in the practice of medicine, would mean the helping of people medically. However, there are various answers to the question of "What is a profession?" One such answer was that a profession could be an occupation or career – an occupation that requires a lot of training and specialized study.

This brief description of a profession suggests to me that a description of surgical pathology would show that changes can and do occur over time (I discussed earlier that my year spent at the New York Hospital in the surgical pathology department under Dr. Arthur Purdy Stout was a great year medically for me, and Dr. Stout was looked up to as a superior teacher for those who wished to practice medicine or surgery.)

Following are some brief discussions from an article published under the title of "The Hospital Laboratory," in the *JAMA* (*Journal of the American Medical Association*) May 23, 1908, over 100 years ago!

Some statements were made in this article that are quite interesting, but changes can and do occur. Was there any justifiable reason for the suggestion to have been recently made to get more trained doctors out into small towns or areas not filled with hospitals? Of course, errors are frequently made, and just because I am obviously opposed to having more doctors sent out to areas other than cities where hospitals exist; that does not mean that I am right and you are wrong.

Several statements from this article, written by an *old* pathologist, follow.

1.) "The rank of the pathologist has been a subordinate one; he has not been appreciated, and the remuneration for his services has been shamefully inadequate."
2.) The pathologist stated that "without pathology help, many medical problems could not be solved."

3.) There were numerous statements made against the pathologist.

Numerous things were brought up here in this 100-year-old medical journal. It just shows what time can do to change various situations. At this time, the pathologist is looked up to in the hospital, and in my former position as Chairman of the Department of Surgery at The Western Pennsylvania Hospital of Pittsburgh, all of the surgical residents were forced to serve a specific time period in the Department of Pathology.

The *American Medical News* of August 11, 2008 (Volume 51 – Number 30) is published by the AMA (American Medical Association) weekly in Chicago, but the contents of articles and expressed opinions are not necessarily endorsed by the AMA. The large heading on the front page of this news volume states in huge letters that hospitals shine light on mistakes by publicly saying: "We're sorry."

Many statements were then written by various individuals and groups about the fact that hospitals and doctors should quite clearly make it known to individuals and various groups when medical and surgical mistakes are made. All kinds of ways to tell everyone who would like to hear about mistakes made by hospital personnel and/or doctors are discussed – but it is quite clear that the "telling of mistakes" should be done by "the other guy – not me."

A number of U.S. states are named and have enacted, "I'm sorry" laws that allow doctors to express sympathy to patients for doctor errors – but the entire description of this "error" problem is just ridiculous to me. The doctor or hospital, whichever, certainly can tell the patient anything about errors – but who may pay the bill? Whenever?

Every effort should be made by doctors and hospitals to prevent errors – but they will continue to occur for one reason or another. The average doctor has his personal opinion about the average lawyer: is money involved in his thinking? But is there any way that a lawyer could help the doctor and not be involved in some fashion that would cost the doctor money? All lawyers are in the legal business not just to attempt to win money in medico-legal situations; and this is shown as follows.

In 1965 Cyril Wecht, MD, JD, was Director of the Institute of Forensic Sciences at Duquesne University School of Law, Pittsburgh, PA.

Cyril has been well known to me personally for many years, as I had been a lecturer in his class at medical school and also in law school. I do not remember how I was invited to talk about surgery in medical school nor law in law school.

Much later, Cyril became coroner of Allegheny County and his department had close relations with me. I initially was Chairman of The Western Pennsylvania Hospital Surgery Department and Burn//Trauma Center in 1970.

There were a number of deaths over the years, so Cyril's department was frequently involved. Cyril also went to extremes when he accepted requests from me, years 1970 to 1990, to speak to my surgical residents about surgery and the law.

In 1965, Cyril designed and began to conduct an unbelievable meeting at Duquesne Law School. That meeting was an unusual course of studies called Post-Graduate Seminars; seminar means "…engaged in original research or intensive study under the guidance of a professor." The name of this course was Law in Medicine, and it was held at Duquesne Law School on an absolutely specific number of hours on specific days from January 6th to March 24th, 1965.

The individuals who had been invited to attend these meetings were doctors and lawyers only; and not one lawyer or doctor ever missed a meeting – it even became difficult to close a meeting at a reasonable time as the lawyers and doctors could not stop discussing this relationship among them.

This is the exact type of meeting that could be carried out today and there would not be any "I'm sorry" type of law. There would just be plain common sense, trained ability and honesty. Following is how these Law in Medicine meetings were carried out.

Cyril Wecht designed this meeting. The lawyers began immediately to promptly think and act as doctors and the doctors as lawyers. The doctors presented their evaluation of a presented medical problem as if they were lawyers and the lawyers had to think like doctors and present arguments in response.

One would have difficulty believing how sincerely the lawyers and doctors argued with each other in their reversed backgrounds. This unusual approach to medico-legal situations was just beyond comprehension. And why was it a complete, acceptable and practical approach to this huge problem? It was an honest technique and there developed a great understanding by the doctors and lawyers for each group's basic evaluation of each specialty.

It is my personal opinion that this described type of meeting between lawyers and medical individuals would be a huge success today. Any reason not to try it?

For the last many years, I have believed that Cyril Wecht has actually done a lot of good for many people. Certainly, Cyril has been outspoken in a variety of ways but most individuals are, in one way or another. It just remains my absolute knowledge that Cyril has done numerous good things for people, although there have always been countless things written about him attempting to prove that he has always been just for himself.

The lawyer-doctor seminar organized and run by Cyril Wecht did a tremendous amount of good for the lawyers and doctors of that 1965 period —and then all kinds of good things for the individuals who sought to work with lawyers and doctors.

It is my personal opinion that a similar type meeting should be run on a yearly basis. But there never was any type of publication – in any medical journal, public article or newspaper – regarding the lawyer and medical doctor relationship that had been thoroughly worked through in 1965.

There are a couple of articles available that discuss the liability problem but it appears to me that doctors of medicine and lawyers are still greatly concerned about money. Money is the real interest for the lawyer, and money is the real interest for the medical man who is trying not to let a lawyer get his money.

The *American Medical News* of February 9, 2009, had a most interesting two-page discussion of mediation as a method to avoid a costly, adversarial court situation. Mediation, to me, does not solve medical patient problems.

Another *American Medical News* of July 28, 2008 really attempts to duck the issues that we had been discussing. In this article, the lawyers presented a made-up case and presented it to about 30 judges who presided over this mock trial.

There is no question about the fact that there exist major problems among patients who appear to have been injured in some medical fashion. Certainly efforts are being made to manage medical patient problems properly. However, it still appears to me that the most straightforward approach to this continued problem is to refer to the Cyril Wecht lawyer-doctor seminar of 1965.

SURGERY – MONEY?

A most interesting article appeared in the *New York Times* on Tuesday, November 27, 2007, about Dr. Michael E. DeBakey and Dr. Denton A. Cooley meeting together after countless years of separation. I have never met Dr. DeBakey, who was 99 years old in 2007, but I had become acquainted with Dr. Cooley, age 87, in San Francisco many years ago.

Years ago, U.S. Steel Company loaned me an airplane and our friend Marcus Aurelius of Fox Chapel was flown to Houston, Texas, for Denton Cooley to operate on Mark's heart. Mark had worked in Pittsburgh at U.S. Steel for many years.

But, the newspaper article could not clearly state what this meeting of the two surgeons was all about in 2007.

How and why did Dr. Cooley steal an artificial heart from Dr. DeBakey—a heart made by DeBakey in 1968 – and then implant it into a patient of his own?

Dr. DeBakey and Dr. Cooley had worked together at the Methodist Hospital for years and then Cooley moved away from that hospital in 1960 where he had worked with DeBakey and set up the Texas Heart Institute at St. Luke's Hospital, several hundred yards from the Methodist Hospital. Both surgeons were said to have had "Texas-size egos."

The *New York Times* newspaper article could not actually determine why these two surgeons met after countless years of separation. It did not look to the reader as if they had become friends again. Dr. DeBakey had made this artificial heart but had never inserted it into a human. Nine years after De Bakey had made this heart, Cooley in some way actually stole it and inserted it into one of his own patients.

Why the meeting of these two surgeons after such a large number of years apart from each other? Following is the *New York Times* answer, in a way.

(Over the years, Dr. DeBakey has called that first-ever use of a total artificial heart a theft, a betrayal, unethical and "a childish act" to claim a medical first. Dr. Cooley defended the implant as a desperate, if ultimately unsuccessful, act to save a life.)

One can here form his or her own opinion. I, for one, agree absolutely with Dr. DeBakey. Might one think money or an act to help an individual?

The *Pittsburgh Tribune-Review* newspaper has done an unbelievable piece of work on publishing factual material on liver transplants. My discussion of liver transplants was not going to be a big item until the very last article on this subject was published May 11, 2008. That caused me to dig up the other articles on liver transplants published by the *Pittsburgh Tribune-Review* on March 9, 10, 21 and 23, 2008; April 20, 2008, and the most recent, May 11, 2008.

It was stated that a countless number of patients have been given liver transplants when they didn't need them and maybe never needed them. Many of these patients could have lived longer without a transplant but when a transplant has been carried out, that patient has an endless situation with the taking of drugs to prevent infections and failure of the liver to survive; resulting in the failure of the patient to survive in the usual manner.

Many of these patients get livers that surgeons in other areas won't use, as those livers are too old or from cadavers where diseases have been present. I am not going into the absolute reasons why and when liver transplants should be done – because I just do not have that type of basic clinical knowledge. I am going to write about what I have read in newspapers and magazines that I personally believe are honest and sincere about their publications. The fact that I am a surgeon should not lead a reader to believe that I may have a superior piece of knowledge about surgery and business.

The University of Pittsburgh and three other centers are using livers that most hospital centers would not use. Even the famous Dr. Thomas Starzl of the University of Pittsburgh (UPMC), said that these livers should not be used on the least sick patient. There are four institutions of the 127 programs that have done half of the 846 transplants since 2005, in non-critical patients. The four are UPMC, Clarian Health in Indianapolis, Mayo Clinic in Jacksonville and Strong Memorial Hospital in Rochester, New York.

There appears to be a universally used numeric score to rate the degree of liver disease. This is known as MELD for Model End-Stage Liver Disease. This score ranges from 6 for the least sick to 40 for the sickest. The newspaper article also states that the less sick – lower MELD – are three times more likely to die within a year if they have a transplant than if they wait. Four liver transplant hospitals have done half of the transplant on low MELD patients since 2005; 102 cases performed by the University of Pittsburgh medical center.

A huge two-page discussion of liver transplants was published Monday, March 10, 2008, by the *Pittsburgh Tribune-Review.* This discussion has to be completely read to become more than just an article. To completely read these brilliantly written pages is a real education. It's an education regarding brilliant surgery but also how a huge amount of money can be made.

One paragraph will be completely copied just to have the reader appreciate the huge business liver transplants represent. This paragraph is found on page A7 of the Tuesday, March 11, 2008 *Pittsburgh Tribune-Review*. This one small section follows.

> Transplants among least ill patients mean big money for medical centers facing increased competition. By doing transplants no one else will do, centers tap into a pool of some 8,900 patients worth an estimated 4 billion dollars in potential charges. They typically get paid the same, no matter how sick the patients are.

The March 23, 2008 *Tribune-Review* article on liver transplants discusses at length the timing for the transplant. This has a lot to do with how well in general the potential receiver of the transplant is when the surgery is performed. There is not complete agreement on this, some surgeons performing transplants considerably earlier than others. And is there a real concern about the timing of a liver transplant? The answer is yes; particularly if the donor liver comes from a live donor. Dr. Mark S. Roberts at UPMC suggested that some centers perform live-donor liver transplants earlier than what might be considered optimal. UPMC performed 12 live-donor liver transplants in patients with MELD scores of 13 or lower in 2007, compared to 23 each in 2006 and 2005. There have been a number of deaths involving live-donor livers and UPMC officials are studying complications in the approximately 160 live-donor liver transplants done there since 2000.

Dr. Amadeo Marcos, UPMC's chief of transplantation since 2004, abruptly resigned five days before the *Pittsburgh Tribune-Review* published the results of a four-month investigation showing that UPMC and other programs perform liver transplants when patients don't need them.

On Tuesday, May 20, 2008, the *Pittsburgh Tribune-Review* described another shocking review and this was about serious lapses at three California organ transplant programs. In 2005 and 2006, it was pointed out that transplant regulators just did not notice problem programs and patients were not protected properly. This regulator group was put into action by Senator C. Grassley, R-Iowa, ranking member of the Senate Finance committee. He said, "I've found too often that changes don't come very fast, sometimes don't come at all."

There is absolutely no question about the fact that transplantation surgery has done and will continue to do great things for human beings. However, everything comes at a price and some transplantation surgery causes more harm than good.

Could money enter into the performing of transplant surgery on occasion?

Will newspapers never cease publishing articles regarding somewhat eye-raising information regarding liver transplants?

Up to this point, we have been talking about the transplant of livers or other organs so that I would just like to talk about one situation, which every one of us will face at one time or another – death! So? What is the cause of death in numerous instances? This can be quite a difficult question to answer under numerous circumstances. The National Center for Health Statistics has 113 cause-of-death classifications – a condensed version of the 8,000 causes acknowledged by the World Health Organization.

There is one physician, Dr. Ned Nicholson, of Edgefield, S.C. whom I have never met nor have read about until somewhat recently – following the death of a personal acquaintance, Senator Strom Thurmond. Senator Thurmond had frequently called me on my hospital office telephone, to ask me about the physical condition of the wife of former General Matthew Bunker Ridgway. Penny and Matt Ridgway lived at 918 West Waldheim Road in Fox Chapel, Pennsylvania, and Franny and I lived next door to Penny and Matt at 910 West Waldheim – three minutes to Pittsburgh, Pennsylvania. General Ridgway died July 26, 1993. (His wife, Penny, died July 19, 1997.)

Senator Thurmond would call my number without the help of a secretary, to ask about Penny but this was of course before Penny died. We would talk at length about Matt Ridgway – always General Ridgway to Senator Thurmond – and we had become friends from a physical time and then later over our personal talks.

Over time, there has always been the question about "the cause of death" when one died and no one knew why that individual had died. Senator Thurmond died at an age near 100 years, and his doctor, Dr. Ned Nicholson, of Edgefield, S. C. quieted those who had an opinion about the cause of death.

Dr. Nicholson coined the cause of death regarding the death of senator Strom Thurmond as "old age due to multiorgan failure." (The bureau of statistics has not challenged this cause of death statement yet according to Dr. Nicholson.)

BIOPRODUCTS

(This is *all* about surgery and money.)

An unusual telephone call came to me in April of 1988 from a Dr. Gerald Klein, who lived in Brunswick, Maine. Dr. Klein wanted to know if I would be interested in working with him and several others on a research project. Dr. Klein had in some way learned that I was part of a Pittsburgh Burn Center and that I had performed some work with the Organogenesis people.

Some of the work done in the past by my surgical group had been published in medical books but I wanted to talk rather specifically about a research project that this Dr. Klein had in mind.

This telephone caller identified himself as a general surgeon, speaking in rather poor English. He then told me that he had developed an enzyme that would liquefy and remove dead tissue and that it was particularly useful in removing the dead skin of third-degree burn patients. He wondered if I would be interested in working with him on a human research project (the enzyme was being made from the stems of pineapples and although I had been acquainted with the pineapple enzyme, Dr. Klein had modified it.) The entire conversation appeared initially to be somewhat ridiculous until Dr. Klein said he already owned a patent on his technology, that Dr. John Burke of Harvard was the only other person working with him, and that they already had FDA approval to operate on 20 human volunteers. That part of the conversation got my attention, and besides that, he was paying for the call.

I told Dr. Klein that yes, I was interested, but that I knew virtually nothing about his enzyme (we had used enzymes in the burn center to soften burn eschars but not to remove dead tissue) and would have to learn more about the technique before I could possibly give him an answer. I knew immediately when he mentioned an association with Dr. John Burke that he was on to something, but I still had to become personally acquainted with the material.

Dr. Klein was a former German World War II paratrooper, but at this time, an American citizen. He had discovered an enzyme in the stems of pineapples that had the capability, when rubbed on fresh burns, to remove the dead skin quickly, painlessly, and eliminate the need for surgery. This would allow minimal burns to heal in a spontaneous manner or promptly prepare the area in more extensive burns for the accepted skin grafting to cover the unhealed areas. The plan seemed interesting to me, but I wanted to become acquainted with the actual technique. Dr. Klein suggested that I fly up to Maine and operate with him, which I agreed to do.

So, in April of 1988, I flew to Portland, Maine, and was met by Dr. Klein's very lady-like nurse secretary. The drive to Brunswick, about thirty miles, was pleasant, but with minimal conversation with my nice young driver. We arrived in Brunswick, but did not stop at the hospital, where I had assumed the surgery would take place. We did stop about a half-mile out in the country and I was welcomed by Dr. and Mrs. Klein, extremely kind and interesting people. The surgery did, in fact, occur – in Dr. Klein's basement with the patient being a thirty-pound pig.

The most interesting part of this rather unusual "research" was that this material did, in fact, work amazingly well. While I was rather skeptical regarding the many medical claims by companies pushing their products, it was obvious to me that this enzyme did what it was claimed to be capable of accomplishing. So, I thought, where do we go from here? Dr. Klein had a ready answer: a meeting in Boston with the surgeon who had previously worked with Dr. Klein on what became known as DEBRIDASE and the company as BIOPRODUCUTS, Dr. John F. Burke. Dr. Burke's name was well known to me. I previously had an appointment to see Dr. Burke at the Massachusetts General Hospital regarding another skin research problem, but upon my arrival at Dr. Burke's office, his secretary informed me that Dr. Burke was out of the country and that she had forgotten to cancel my appointment. Dr. Burke was Professor of Surgery at Harvard, head of a burn center in Boston, and was internationally known as a surgeon.

(I learned from the driver of the car, as we left the airport at Portland, that Dr. Klein had been a paratrooper in the German army in World War II, was 71 years old, and a fine man. She said his practice was small, he had suffered a stroke two years previously, made very little money, and when he couldn't afford her monthly salary, she just worked for him for nothing.)

On May 31, 1988, I flew to Boston again and meandered over to the Massachusetts General Hospital for my meeting with Dr. Burke and Dr. Klein.

It became quite apparent that Bioproducts needed two things: (1) the use of a burn center to carry out additional clinical trials of their product (Debridase), and (2) a company to financially underwrite them in bringing a product to market. Since a company (Bioproducts) did exist with a number of stockholders, but no income, financing further work was a very acute consideration.

The FDA, as noted previously, had given Bioproducts permission to perform ten operations on humans, burn patients who had to have dead skin removed. Dr. Burke had performed four such procedures and Dr. Klein three. (I'm sure other cases were carried out in various ways on patients with leg ulcers, bedsores, and burns.) I was asked to do three burn cases, to which I agreed. Bioproducts was the sole owner of several patents protecting the Debridase product.

Complicating factors did exist, such as Bioproducts depended on a single Chinese from Taiwan to produce the material from the pineapple stems, since stems from Taiwan purportedly were the best.

I felt comfortable with the proposal arrangements and returned to Pittsburgh that day, prepared to become involved with clinical cases. Approval for me to proceed was granted by the West Penn Institutional Review board (IRB), and arrangements were made promptly for Dr. Klein to fly to Pittsburgh to work with me on several burn patients.

Acceptable cases were chosen, and Dr. Klein and I operated on them. In my opinion, the results were excellent – far better than anything else on the market, which included the well-known Travase enzyme. The next step was to decide how to approach another drug company for financial backing. We were positive the FDA would require that many more clinical cases be done.

I then made arrangements to fly to Boston, find a hotel, and keep a previously arranged meeting with Dr. John Burke.

While walking over to the Massachusetts General Hospital from my hotel, I had to wonder about meeting with the famous Dr. "Jack" Burke. Dr. Burke was retired from his position as Chairman of the Department of Surgery at the Massachusetts General Hospital, but still actively involved in surgery. He had published almost 300 surgical papers – a phenomenal accomplishment.

Meeting Dr. Burke was a true experience (as Dr. Klein and three others were there for this meeting.) He was most impressive and very gentlemanly, while at the same time being quite dogmatic and domineering. Those present were the four men who were the company, Bioproducts, who made all the decisions that controlled the company. There was Dr. Gerald Klein, the surgeon who discovered the enzyme (escharase), which was the active enzyme in the pineapple stem; Dan Lord, former Secretary-Treasurer of L.L. Bean Company in Maine; Dr. Jack Hauch (PhD), a chemist from Seattle, Washington, who just happened to be the one who arranged with a young Chinese woman in Taiwan to obtain pineapple stems; and Dr. Burke. My question, of course, was how the group saw my involvement.

Just a note about the famous Taiwanese enzyme. One morning, I was having coffee with Dr. Klein at his home and the telephone rang. The caller was head of the drug company that made Travase and offered to merge Travase with Debridase and split the huge amount of money that this would bring about. Dr. Klein just said that he was not interested and hung up the telephone. Terrible decision? Yes!

At one time, Roy McKnight, Chairman and CEO for Mylan Laboratories, was somewhat interested in becoming involved with Organogenesis. For that reason, I brought the enzyme work to his attention. He was initially sufficiently interested that he, Patricia Sunseri (Senior Vice-President for Mylan), and I flew to Brunswick, Maine, in October of 1989 so that they could meet Dr. Klein and review the possibility of financial help from Mylan. It was decided that further talks might take place and decisions be reached regarding involvement by Mylan in developing production of the pineapple stem enzyme. A lot of work followed.

Discussion had been proceeding during the spring of 1990 between Bioproducts personnel and Mylan Lab. Drs. Burke, Klein and Hauch, along with Mr. Lord and myself, met in Pittsburgh with the Mylan leaders, and Mylan agreed to investigate thoroughly the work of Bioproducts. It was decided that Bioproducts should carry out more clinical cases with the debriding enzyme, but this couldn't occur in the United States, as the ten cases allotted by the FDA had already been completed. Discussions occurred regarding foreign countries and since Dr. Burke, Dr. Klein and I were relatively well acquainted with Israeli cities and individual doctors there, we decided to make the necessary plans to go there. A major problem arose immediately; it was illegal to take any medical material out of the United States for the purpose of carrying out research in a foreign country. However, taking 90% out and developing or finishing off the remaining 10% was legal. Therefore, we rented a laboratory in Berlin, and Dr. Jack Hauch went there and completed the enzyme product (experience was important here because formulae have been stolen by giving them to an unknown to make up). In the meantime, letters and numerous telephone calls to Israel solidified plans for all of us to go to Israel and work. We decided that we should plan to operate on 15 to 20 burn cases in Israel and that we probably could accomplish that within a two-week period. One major problem was how to convince the Israel authorities to permit us to carry 30 jars of a white ointment from Germany into Israel without opening them (to unscrew a cap on the ointment jar would contaminate the material). But how were they to know that these jars wouldn't explode and kill? The material was carried into Israel by Dr. Klein, and to this day, I'm not sure how he did it.

June 14, 1990

Dr. John C. Gaisford, M.D.
Administration Dep.
West Penn Hospital
4800 Friendship Avenue
Pittsburgh, PA 15224
U.S.A.

Dear Dr. Gaisford,

Prof. Penchas has brought to my attention your letter to him of June 6, 1990, regarding the studies in Israel to determine the efficacy of a Debridase in removing burn eschar.

Prof. Penchas and myself will be very happy to meet you during your stay in Israel and to assist you in collaboration with the group in Hadassah.

As I understand from Dr. A. Eldad of our Dept. of Plastic Surgery, he has already discussed Hadassah's participation in this study with Dr. L. Rosenberg of Beer-Sheva.

Please let me know when it will be possible to meet you and I will do my best to arrange a meeting with Prof. Penchas and Dr. Eldad.

My direct telephone numbers are: Office: 972-2-446095
972-2-437550
Home: 972-2-810682
Fax: 972-2-434434

Looking forward to hearing from you.

Sincerely,

Dr. Avi Treves
Division of Research & Development

cc: Prof. S. Penchas, General Director
Dr. A. Eldad, Dep. of Plastic Surgery
Prof. M. Wexler, Head, Dep. of Plastic Surgery

John C. Gaisford, M.D.

Mellon Pavilion Suite 340
4815 Liberty Avenue
Pittsburgh, PA 15224

Telephone
(412) 681-5266

June 20, 1990

Avi Treves, M.D.
Hadassah Medical Organization
P.O.B. 12000
Jerusalem, Israel

Dear Dr. Treves:

Thank you for your kind letter, which I received yesterday. My plans are to arrive in Tel Aviv this Sunday and meet with Drs. Rosenberg, Klein, and Burke at the airport. From there we will drive to Beer Sheva.

I will call you promptly and discuss available meeting times.

Thank you again and kindest regards.

Sincerely,

Jack Gaisford

John C. Gaisford, M.D.

JCG/kas

LETTER TO ISRAEL

Through our personal contacts in Israel, our plan was to do this work at a hospital in Beer Sheva. Dr. Ilor Rosenberg, a well-known plastic surgeon with a very large practice in that hospital, agreed to work with us. Therefore, arrangements were made for all of us to meet in the Tel Aviv airport on June 24, 1990 at 3:00 PM. Dr. Klein and Dan Lord would be arriving from Germany, Dr. Burke from Boston, and I from New York City (obviously on three separate schedules).

I immediately needed airline reservations, and wanted El Al, thinking it was the safest. Not being able to get transportation that way, I obtained TWA tickets (business class) at a cost of $3,363. The flights from

Pittsburgh to Tel Aviv were extremely uninteresting, but physically debilitating (left Pittsburgh Saturday, June 23, at 2:00 PM; left New York at 6:00 PM; arrived at Tel Aviv International about noon on Sunday, June 24).

The Tel Aviv airport is a most busy place – and big! I had nothing to do for three hours – or so I thought. Between noon and 5:00 PM, there were two bomb alerts, when every person was forced to run as fast as he could from the airport building to surrounding fields or parking lots. Fortunately, both alarms were false, but somewhat unnerving. Several hours passed; I managed to buy some kind of a soft drink, read a little, and got more tired. When 5:00 PM arrived and there was no sign of my various cohorts, I knew I either had to find a Tel Aviv hotel or find my way to Beer Sheba (Beer Sheva is Israeli spelling). I decided to hire a taxi to take me to Beer Sheva, 75 miles down the only road in that direction. I located the Desert Inn and went to bed. The others arrived about 10:00 PM.

Everyone showed up and I met them early in the morning. We took a ten-minute taxi ride to the hospital where we were to work, the Seroka Hospital, part of the Ben-Gurion University of the Negev. We had already set in place our surgical plans with the Director of the Plastic Surgery Service at Seroka, Dr. Ilor Rosenberg. Surgery arrangements had been previously made, so that on our first full day in Beer Sheva, we operated on four patients. During our stay, the patient mix was somewhat different: Jews, Palestinians and Bedouins. Not only were the patients interesting, but the protection policy was unbelievable. Heavily armed Israeli soldiers roamed every floor constantly, and were doubly certain that only the proper people entered the operating rooms. Incidentally, this work was in June and July in the Negev Desert in a non-air-conditioned hospital. Even the hotel was without air-conditioning.

My room was on the second floor, but a door to the outside could not be closed snugly, and that part of the hotel faced a grove of trees. I pushed a heavy chest of drawers against the door, thinking it might help in preventing an intruder from entering my room.

The work progressed well; it was well documented by tapes, photographs and discussions among us. The patients appeared to appreciate our work, particularly the Bedouins. More plans were made for daily surgery, but also for some geographic trips. The schedule may make it appear as if this was vacation time, but the very nature of our surgery (applying our enzyme material sometimes at noon, and then waiting four and sometimes eight hours to operate made for huge time lapses, allowing time for side trips.)

VISITING SCHEDULE: DEBRIDASE II 24-6 / 3-7-90

24-6-90	1515 + 1900	LANDING IN TEL-AVIV (Lior welcomes & clears Customs & Immigration)
	2230	ARRIVAL TO THE "DESERT INN", BEER SHEVA, GOOD NIGHT
25-6-90	0800	MORNING ROUNDS, PATIENT SORTING & TREATMENT.
	1300	LUNCHEON-RECEPTION, SMALL DINNING ROOM (Med. School dean, University R & D dean, Hospital director, hospital administrator, 7 chiefs of divisions, department staff)
	1600	PRESENTATION OF "DEBRIDASE" TO THE SURGICAL DIVISION MEDICAL STAFF. (Press conference will follow)
	----	FREE EVENING TO RELAX.
26-6-90	0800	MORNING ROUNDS, CLINICAL & RESEARCH ACTIVITY
	2000	DINNER AT Lior's HOME
	10:00	Visit to the University Campus.
27-6-90	0600	TOUR TO MASSADA, DEAD-SEA, EIN GEDI & THE RECONSTRUCTED ANCIENT TOWN OF SUSSIA - (Visitors) (Clinical & Research continue - Lior)
28-6-90	0700	TOUR OF THE BEDOUIN MARKET
	0830	MORNING ROUNDS, CLINICAL & RESEARCH ACTIVITY (Lior).
	0900	TOUR TO THE INSTITUTE OF DESERT RESEARCH & SDE BOKER.
29-6-90 Friday	0800	MORNING ROUNDS, CLINICAL & RESEARCH ACTIVITY
		Evening leaving for Tel Aviv (Clinical & Research continue - Lior)
30-6-90 Sat	0700	TOUR OF GALLILE, NAZARET ETC.
		Night in Tel Aviv (Clinical & Research continue - Lior)
1 -7-90 Sun	0630	TOUR OF JERUSALEM (Visitors) (Clinical & Research continue - Lior)
		Evening BACK TO BEER SHEVA
2 -7-90 Mon	0800	MORNING ROUNDS, CLINICAL & RESEARCH ACTIVITY
	2000	FAREWELL DINNER
3 -7-90 Tues	0500	DEPARTURE FOR AIRPORT
	0800	MORNING ROUNDS, CLINICAL & RESEARCH ACTIVITY (of the remaining team until program is ended).

* THE PROJECT WILL PROCEED REGARDLESS OF TOURS, DINNERS, ORGIES ETC.
* REMOUNT WORKS ARE IN COURSE IN THE DEPARTMENT, SORRY FOR THE MESS.
* 6 ROOMS RESERVED IN RESPECTIVE DAYS IN BEER SHEVA & TEL AVIV

This was a schedule that was arranged for us, if we wished to follow it, as there were hours from the time that we had applied the escarase until we could surgically remove the burned areas.

It had not been thoroughly discussed, previous to our trip to Israel, that Dr. Klein had determined that it was necessary to wait six to eight hours after the enzyme had been applied before an attempt was made to remove the burned skin of a patient. Another situation existed that may prevent the use of the enzyme material, and that was that the usual drugs (such as even penicillin) could not be used during the time period between application of the enzymes and the attempted removal of the burned tissue. Dr. Klein had not brought that to my attention – had he told the others, including Mylan?

(Not every day was spent in the operating room.) A swim in the Dead Sea was a unique experience. The water is 1300 feet below sea level, and the salt content so great that it is physically impossible to sink. The salt in the water looks like huge blocks of ice in the Allegheny River on a cold winter day. The Dead Sea yields vast amounts of bromine and potash with bromine burns being quite common – we operated on two bromine-type burns. It was a strange feeling that existed when a glance east showed the rugged mountains of Jordan bordering that side of the Dead Sea. (Dr. Jack Burke, the famous Harvard professor, shared the Dead Sea with me.)

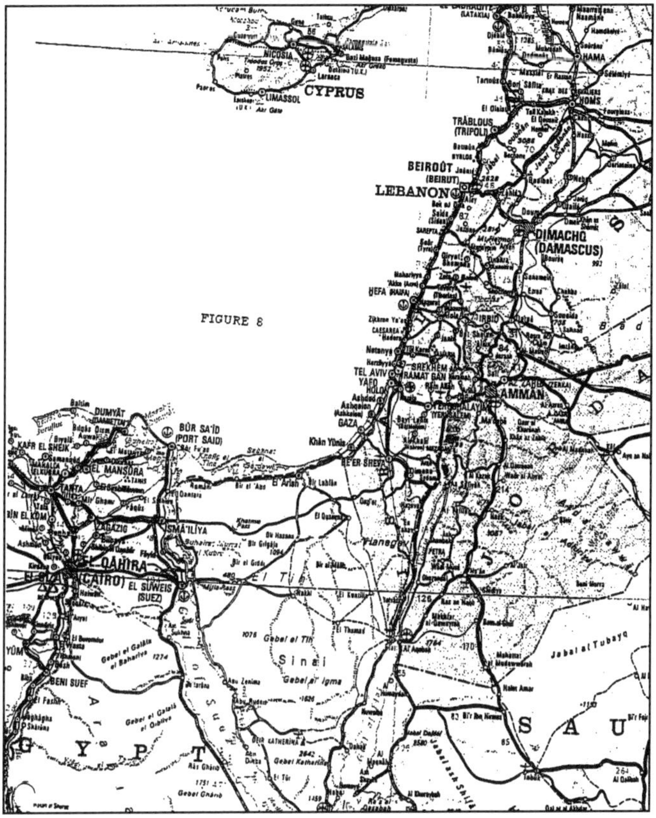

An interesting map of Israel.

Dr. Arieh Eldad headed the Burn Center at Hadassah and was most interesting. He wanted to see the operation I was scheduled to perform that afternoon in Beer Sheva, and offered to drive me there from Jerusalem. He had an old worn-out car, and suggested we save 30 minutes on the 80-mile trip by driving the West Bank through Hebron. He said we probably would be stoned, but the Palestinians there had no guns. With that, he pulled up the back seat to reveal an automatic rifle. My answer to that was to take the other road toward Tel Aviv and forget Hebron as the operation would not take place until we got there anyhow.

For some years, it has been thought that Israel was attempting to build an atom bomb. Material (uranium) used in making such a bomb had certainly disappeared some time previously on the high seas, and Israel was the suspected hijacker. When driving south to Beer Sheva, Dr. Eldad pointed out an area to me where the entrance was quite heavily guarded and where he thought the bomb might be housed. Attached is information regarding this so-called nuclear plant from the thriller "Triple" and the *London Daily Telegraph* of May 7, 1977.

TRIPLE

"A LITERALLY EARTH-SHAKING CONFRONTATION!" —*The New York Times*

" A REAL PAGE-TURNER...PACED WITH A RACING HEARTBEAT FOR A METRONOME!" —*Boston Globe*

EGYPT—where, hidden deep in the desert, a top-secret project to build a nuclear plant that will give the Arabs "the bomb" nears completion...

ISRAEL—where the Mossad's number-one agent, Nat Dickstein, a master of disguise and deceit, is given the impossible mission: to beat the Arabs in the nuclear arms race by finding and stealing 200 tons of uranium without any other nation discovering the theft...

RUSSIA—where top KGB officials have decided to tip the atomic balance in Egypt's favor...

ENGLAND—where Dickstein makes what could be the fatal mistake of his career by falling under the seductive spell of Suza Ashford, the dazzling, dark-haired beauty who may be his dearest ally or deadliest enemy...

THE HIGH SEAS—where the Mossad, KGB, Egyptians, and Fedayeen terrorists play out the final violent, bloody moves in this devastating game where the price of failure is nuclear holocaust...

POSTSCRIPT

From the *London Daily Telegraph* of May 7, 1977:

ISRAEL SUSPECTED OF HIJACKING SHIP WITH URANIUM

by Henry Miller in New York

Israel is believed to have been behind the disappearance from the high seas nine years ago a uranium shipment large enough to build 30 nuclear weapons, it was disclosed yesterday.

Officials say that the incident was "a real James Bond affair" and that although intelligence agencies in four countries investigated the mystery, it was never determined what had actually happened to the 200 tons of uranium ore that vanished...

—Quoted by permission of The Daily Telegraph, Ltd.

Following is a bit of information on the hospital area where we had done all our surgery. Our work proved that the pineapple enzyme really did work as a non-surgical method for removing burned skin.

Ben-Gurion University of the Negev

Ben-Gurion University of the Negev is a unique and pioneering institution of higher learning. Inspired by the vision and lofty aspirations of Israel's foremost statesman, the late David Ben-Gurion, the University was established in 1969 and charged with a vital mandate — to spearhead the development of the Negev, Israel's vast desert area.

Today, Ben-Gurion University, with campuses in Beer-Sheva and Sede Boqer, is a major center of education and research in Israel. Moreover, the University has played a leading role in establishing new industry and thriving communities in the Negev. Ben-Gurion University awards degrees in the principal academic fields. Undergraduates and graduate students may choose from a wide array of courses in the Faculties of Natural Sciences, Engineenng Sciences, Humanities and Social Sciences, and Health Sciences. The School for Continuing Education provides numerous adult education courses for the public at large.

We did our work at the Beer-Sheva campus of Ben-Gurion University of the Negev. This university hospital was superb—advanced in every degree. The pineapple stem burn treatment project was completed without any difficulties. And then, after becoming quite well acquainted with the West Bank, Gaza, the Dead Sea and the Negev Desert, we returned to the United States.

I spent July 4, 1990 at the Sheraton Hotel by the Mediterranean Sea in Tel Aviv. On July 5th, I boarded a TWA flight, presumably to refuel in Paris and then fly non-stop to New York. Things didn't quite work out that way. An air controller strike began that day in Paris, so we had to fly to Switzerland to re-fuel. All New York passengers went through United States customs in Switzerland (I had no knowledge that such a thing could be done), which took hours.

Finally, we were rolling down the runway when the captain came on to report that since this runway was quite short, a full load of fuel could not be taken on and another re-fueling stop would be necessary before crossing the Atlantic. So – we stopped in Ireland. (I didn't even look out to see where we had landed in Ireland.) After quite some time, we were in the air again.

We reached New York about 10:00 PM; I caught a flight on some airline to Pittsburgh, and in some way got home after another impossible number of hours, early on July 6, 1990.

After returning to Pittsburgh in 1990 and delivering the results of our work in Israel to the Mylan corporation, most of us believed that we had certainly proven that our work regarding a new technique for the treatment of burns would be put promptly to use across the country, assuming that the FDA would listen to us and make it possible for Mylan to obtain a patent.

So why bother to have discussed this "pineapple juice" burn treatment over the last number of pages? Doesn't this appear to have been an extremely long run for such a short slide? No, I don't think so. Yes, it was not only a long run but a very expensive one. Mylan was never able to obtain a patent permitting us to use this material, and we have never treated a burn case with this enzyme since the last case we treated in

Israel in 1990. And how many millions of dollars did Mylan Laboratories use and lose in working with us? Too many.

This was a fair description of so-called clinical trials. But in many instances it takes several years to complete such work adequately.

While there was marked disappointment by all involved that a patent to use this pineapple drug could not be obtained, everyone did not quit working. I personally was invited by the Mylan Corporation to become involved in other medical projects. Roy McKnight called me by telephone one night. He bluntly stated that I had personally carried out much work on behalf or Mylan – numerous flights to Brunswick to work on pigs, all of the operations on burn patients at the West Penn Burn/Trauma Center using the pineapple material, the extensive trip and work in Israel – and that I was a poor business man and had never sent a bill to Mylan for all of my work. Therefore, he was calling to invite me to become a member of the Mylan Board of Directors. I maintained that position for eight years.

Roy McKnight died in November of 1993, while sitting at an evening Board of Directors Meeting at the Indian Creek Golf Club in Florida. Mylan lost a great leader and I lost a good friend.

10 || INTERESTING PEOPLE & COMPANIES

Every individual knows about people and companies that were interesting or who clearly helped other people. Was this read in the morning paper, witnessed whatever the nice thing was, or seen on the evening television program? Unfortunately, that which was seen or read about is generally forgotten rather promptly.

The author has been involved in various manners with some of these interesting individuals and companies and will discuss them as follows.

ALCOA

December 19, 1979, a few days before Christmas, appeared to be just another December day, until the telephone rang about 6:00 PM. The Medical Director of the Alcoa Corporation was calling, wanting to know if there would be someone available to see, examine and care for a man who worked for Alcoa and had been badly burned. My answer of course was "yes," but I was informed that a trip would be necessary. I promptly said that I myself would handle that burn problem, thinking that the trip might be to Turtle Creek or even Monongahela. The trip? Suriname, previously Dutch Guiana in South America, adjacent to Brazil.

The Alcoa spokesman said that an Alcoa Lear Jet and Alcoa's two senior pilots would be available for this long trip. My wife just blinked her eyes a couple of times – possibly accepting certain peculiar things her doctor husband did – but made no attempt at asking me to have someone else treat that burn victim. I did not know at that time that the largest business in Suriname was the Alcoa Corporation.

Before hanging up on that initial telephone call, I asked the Alcoa Medical Director if I might ask the head nurse of the Burn/Trauma Center, Karen Price, to make the trip with me, and the answer, of course, was yes.

Karen was living with her mother and father and answered my call, which was then about seven in the evening. The request for her to meet at the Allegheny Country Airport at 8:00 AM the next morning was answered by – "I'll be there." And she was not late, accompanied by her mother and dad. Karen had been well informed about the nature of the trip, as I had called her and explained the circumstances.

The flight to Suriname was uneventful, and we reached the one and only airport in that country about four in the afternoon. The airport was 35 miles from Paramaribo, the capital of Suriname

We were met by Dr. L.E. Olmtak, the Medical Director at Suralco (Alcoa), and we were taken directly to the hospital where the Alcoa burn victim lay.

The patient was an extremely large black man with serious, life-threatening burns. Karen and I knew exactly what decisions had to be made immediately. There was one obvious major fact – if we elected to treat this man in Paramaribo, it would mean a 7-10 day stay. There were no doctors in that city who could keep this man alive. The alternative was to attempt to get him on our jet and return him to the West Penn Hospital Burn Unit. Certainly we knew that Christmas was just around the corner, but that fact did not really enter into the decision that was made, that being to attempt to get a huge unconscious man onto a stretcher and into that Lear Jet. The decision was made – back to Pittsburgh!

The following morning, December 21, we had this man at the airport. The Leer Jet door had been measured, and we knew then that the stretcher could make it through.

And there on the ground, just steps away from the plane's steps, were our patient's pretty black wife and their three young children, standing absolutely straight, arms at their sides, tears streaming down their cheeks, possibly seeing a live husband and father for the last time.

This man had excellent care on that trip back to the United States. He was in and out of consciousness, but survived. Because of the position of the stretcher and a large amount of equipment, the toilet was blocked, and for some strange reason, the pilots had to find an island for a 10-minute stop.

We reached Pittsburgh late that afternoon, and the patient was taken by helicopter to the West Penn Hospital Burn Center. This man did extremely well, having very extensive skin grafts, and it was only two months later that he was fitted with American clothes and flown back to Suriname to be with his family – and his job with Alcoa.

Alcoa's involvement in Suriname? Alcoa is the largest business in that country, employing over 5,000 Surinamese. But this was not the end of the story. With the same pilots and the same jet, plus one wife, one more doctor and two Burn Center nurses, the return trip to Suriname began our teaching in the medical school at Paramaribo. What Alcoa did for countless people there was indescribably wonderful.

The burned man from Suriname had numerous Alcoa Corporation visitors at the West Penn Burn Center. Very quickly the head nurse, Karen, was asked many questions about interns, residents, and other nurses. Obviously, there was discussion among the Alcoa people regarding how some of this teaching could be carried out at the University of Suriname by West Penn Hospital doctors and nurses.

The Alcoa Corporation offered an invitation to several professionals associated with the West Penn Burn Center to go to Suriname and help teach at Suriname University (Universiteit van Suriname).

This Alcoa invitation was promptly discussed among us, and a decision was made as to those who would be involved. They were Karen Price, head nurse of the Burn Center; Doreen Konop, the assistant head nurse; Harvey Slater, MD, who worked with me and later became Director of the Burn Center; and my wife, Frances.

The same Alcoa jet and pilots flew this group to Suriname on August 2, 1980. All of our teaching plans had been coordinated among us so that we were prepared to do what was expected of us.

The evening of August 2 was more than a little unusual. We were guests of the Dean of the Medical School of Suriname University, Professor Dr. F. Jessurun. As noted in the list of some of those at this dinner party, it was an unusual group. One particular incident occurred involving our American Ambassador, Mr. Jack

Crowley. The drinks that were served must have seemed quite good to one of us as I overhead Doreen Konop call our Ambassador by his first name.

Parmiribo – 02: August 1980
Universiteit van Suriname

Dr. Jack Tjong Tjin Joe (Minister of Health)	Herman Snastraat 25 Paramariba-Suriname
Mr. Jack Crowley (American Ambassador)	c/o American Embassy Dr. S. Redmondstraat 11-13 Paramaribo-Suriname
Dr. John Hewitt (Surgeon)	Andirastraat pc. 17 Ultvlugt – Suriname
Prof. Dr. F. Jessurun (Dean of the Medical School)	c/o M.W.I. Kernkampweg 3 Paramaribo – Suriname
Mr. Leonard Jacob, Jr. (Managing Director Suralco)	c/o Suralco Kendall Br. P.O. Box 560343 Miami, FL 33156 USA

cc: Dr. L.E. Olmtak
Medical Director – Suralco

The above were dinner partners for this group from The Western Pennsylvania Hospital Burn/Trauma Center, Pittsburgh, Pennsylvania.

The Medical School was a beautiful school, and the West Penn Burn Center speakers attempted to make their long trip to South America meaningful. The lecture hours were somewhat unusual, but everything worked out well.

Following are schedules for the days and hours of our talks.

SURINAME BURN SYMPOSIUM

August 3, 4, 5, 1980

Sunday, August 3, 1980	**9:00 AM – 1:30 PM**
9:00 – 9:30 AM	Introduction of West Penn Hospital Faculty Introduction of the Burn Problem JOHN C. GAISFORD, MD
9:30 – 10:00 AM	Outpatient Burn Treatment HARVEY SLATER, M.D.
10:00 – 10:30 AM	Management of the Burn Patient in a General Hospital Setting KAREN PRICE, RN
10:30 – 11:00 AM	Establishment of a Burn Center JOHN C. GAISFORD, MD
11:00 – 11:30 AM	COFFEE BREAK
11:30 – NOON	Pre-Hospital Burn Care KAREN PRICE, RN
NOON – 12:30 PM	Nursing Care in a Burn Unit DOREEN KONOP, RN
12:30 – 1:00 PM	Fluids and Antibiotics HARVEY SLATER, MD

Monday August 4, 1980	8:00 –10:30 PM
8:00 – 8:30 PM	Electrical Burns HARVEY SLATER MD
8:30 – 9:00 PM	Nursing Care for Burned Children KAREN PRICE RN
9:00 – 9:30 PM	Psychological Problems of the Burned Patient DOREEN KONOP, RN
9:30 – 10:00 PM	Burns of the Genitalia
10:00 – 10:30 PM	Film on Skin Grafting Film on Pressure Garments JOHN C GAISFORD MD
Tuesday August 5, 1980	**8:00 – 10:30 PM**
8:00 – 8:30 PM	Medical Complications in the Burned Patient (Renal, pulmonary, hypertension, etc.) HARVEY SLATER, MD
8:30 – 9:00 PM	Nutrition DOREEN KONOP, RN
9:00 – 9:30 PM	Physical and Occupational Therapy KAREN PRICE, RN
9:30 – 10:00 PM	Early Excision and Immediate Skin Grafting HARVEY SLATER, MD
10:00 – 10:30 PM	Reconstructive Procedures JOHN C. GAISFORD MD

This group was shown countless interesting parts of the city of Paramaribo, but, in addition, several trips were made outside of the city that were unbelievably educational.

This rather odd group of West Penn Hospital Burn/Trauma individuals was asked if we would like to see another part of Suriname before we returned to Pittsburgh. Obviously, we all promptly said that we would be delighted – and the trip from the capital of the country, Paramaribo, was outstanding.

We were flown on a relatively small airplane to a section of Suriname with a huge lake. During our flight one of the local doctors described what we were going to be involved in – a fishing trip. He then told us that we would be taken in small boats out into this so-called lake to fish for piranhas. These fish were the only ones in that piece of water because these piranhas would not allow another fish to exist. They killed the others. Piranhas were, on average, seven inches long, had a number of rows of dagger-like teeth, and were known to be able to physically destroy these humans if they dared to attempt to swim in that so-called lake. At this point, Dr. Slater turned a little green and voiced his desire not to go fishing. He did, however, agree to give it a brief, careful try.

The lake was huge. It was really spectacular, as there were countless tiny islands dotted everywhere, some with a few yards of ground and one or two trees. It demanded a discussion about all of what we were seeing, and we were promptly and completely apprised of the sight.

Because Alcoa was so huge, employing 5,000 local natives and with no other piece of big business in Suriname, but a demand by Alcoa for power, the Suriname River had been damned, creating this huge lake. And what it had done was to have covered countless acres of land with water, stranding countless animals of every size and description with nowhere to go. They faced death by starvation or drowning. And this brought forth a fantastic story about a Pittsburgher who came to the rescue of countless animals.

Mrs. Sarah Mellon Scaife of Pittsburgh gave a huge amount of money to Suriname in an effort to save as many of these animals as possible, by taking them off these tiny islands and placing them on dry land. This is just one more instance of what a human being can do for others. Did any of this ever appear in a Pittsburgh newspaper? Possibly.

Well, the fishing in this huge man-made lake went well. Harvey Slater did not get wet, he caught a few piranhas, but had the driver of his motorboat remove the hook each time from the mouth of his caught fish.

Personally, I just got a little bit wet, but had no piranha problems. The small motor boat in which I was riding went south to the end of the country, and just before this boat met up with land, I asked to have the boat stopped, got off and put one foot on land – Brazil. It was then honest for me to say that I had been in that country – Brazil.

The flight from Suriname back to Pittsburgh was without incident. We had been invited to return for further teaching, and received a nice letter from Dr. Olmtak of Alcoa shortly after our return home.

FROM : L.E. Olmtak
Paramaribo

TO : Mr.J. Yates
Pittsburgh

1980-08-08

The Burn Symposium given by Dr.John Gaisford and his co workers from the Burn Unit of the West Penn Hospital has been an enormous succes.
Attendance was more than 100%, and all presentations were well received and highly appreciated.

In general the people at our University were very impressed and their opinion was that this symposium was one of the best we ever had, not only because the team was so well prepared on the subject but also because they all appear to be such very fine persons.

Also on behalf of the Medical Faculty of our University I wish to express our sincerest appreciation and gratitude for your support to make these experts available to Suriname.

L.E. Olmtak

cc. Mr.L. Jacob -Pbo
Dr.J. Gaisford-Pgh

BOB PRINCE

There probably was no other man in Pittsburgh who was as well known and well liked as Bob Prince. Did I like him?— He was one of my patients and I never had a nicer one. Bob was the one who knew how to broadcast the Pirates ballgames and that made everyone who owned a radio listen to him. However, there was a game other than baseball where Bob did so much for kids. (Bob had a kid of his own who needed help and he got it.) This special game – the Ham Am. And Bob Prince started this special game!

The Ham AM – what was it? The name "Ham" was used to describe the individual who may like to play golf but who knew less than nothing about the game – so, he was a terrible player. The word "AM" was coined to be short for "Amateur." And, therefore, the "HAM AM" was a Dumb Amateur Tournament. Bob Prince brought the Ham Am into existence and ran it with a tight fist.

It cost each player who arrived to play in the Ham Am so many dollars. (My memory is not very good just now, but I believe it was ten dollars.) Many gave Bob more than ten when the individuals realized that all the money paid to play would at the end of the day go to a college caddie fund.

But – who would decide which caddy would get the money and/or how much would go to whomever? Bob Prince made all the rules and regulations associated with the Ham Am. No doubt the most important aspect of this golf event was that the caddies would profit. Bob decided that caddies who absolutely wanted to go to college but had no financial backing of any kind, would be helped.

There was another group of so-called golfers, a group who did not play golf at all, who would come to the club where the Ham Am was to be played and contribute a few dollars just to help the caddie fund — and then have a drink?

This caddie fund really and truly helped a number of caddies as they actually ended up in college. To my knowledge, it was never determined who picked the caddies who were to receive this money. Everybody clearly trusted Bob Prince in absolutely every way.

And then Bob died! How was the Ham Am then to be run? This tournament began to end after Bob was gone. There was less and less money placed into the so-called caddie-for-college fund, as this money appeared just to be used for whatever expenses that existed just to run the event.

What else happened to this popular Ham Am golf event? The Ham Am one year did not appear on the yearly golf schedule – it just disappeared!

But all the individuals who ever attended the Ham Am day golf tournament will never forget Bob Prince. He truly helped a lot of caddies, who had no money, get to college!

SIMON HAFNER & BEN PAUL BRASELY
(AND THEIR COLLEGE STUDENTS)

Simon Hafner was a personal friend of mine for many years. He had come to the United States when he was nine years old and never even graduated from high school. His original home was Russia. Simon developed his own business but became a millionaire by way of the stock market.

Ben Paul Brasely was a close friend of Simon's. Mr. Brasely was an extremely well-known Pittsburgh lawyer and a true gentleman.

These two men had no children but were wealthy and desired to help others. They wanted to help a number of children go to college, by paying for everything. They asked me to choose individuals for them, having given me instructions. They did not care whether the young person was black or white, Jew, Gentile or of any other group. The boy or girl had to be from a family that did not have money available to send a child to college.

They depended upon me to evaluate potential college material and it was up to me to offer what there was to be. I would be the individual who would explain to the college student–to-be in detail how these plans would be carried out.

There was one absolute decision handed to me and that was that none of these kids whom I chose for college were ever to learn who was behind all their college expenses.

This was one of the most difficult jobs that I had ever experienced but I thanked Simon and Ben Paul for having chosen me.

I kept these two great men, Simon and Ben Paul, up-to-date regarding the chosen individuals.

My personal opinion was that what these two had done was the greatest experience in which I had ever been involved.

And the chosen college individuals? They kept thanking me for carrying their thanks to whomever was behind such unusual, great work.

ANDREW MORRISON

There are many things that happen on golf courses, some being somewhat funny, peculiar, or unacceptable. At other times, it's business, making/losing money on bets, or peculiar accidents. And then there are instances when extremely nice situations occur, one which could never be forgotten by those who witnessed this one or read the following story.

Andrew J. Morrison is a member of the Fox Chapel Golf Club and a personal friend. He loves golf and is a basically good player. However, there are days when the weather is perfect for those who plan to play golf but choose to use their available time to do something else.

This short, but extremely interesting and beautiful story, involves Andrew and his wheel-chair-bound son.

This little kid – about 10 years old? – could not get out of his wheelchair. He could not walk, but his dad was seen by me and obviously many others, pushing his boy from the Fox chapel Clubhouse about 350 yards over to the practice putting green and practice fairway. And was Andrew taking his little boy who could not even walk over to the golf practice area – just so he, the dad, could hit balls and fulfill the job of managing his young wheelchair-bound son? No - Andrew took his young wheelchair-bound son over to the club's golf practice area to help his son swing golf clubs and hit golf balls. And right here is where I voted to make Andrew the real golfing victor! He taught his boy how to swing his golf clubs and hit golf balls.

I witnessed this very unusual young golfer swinging a club and actually hitting good shots. On more than one occasion, I spent short periods of time with Andrew and his son just to watch this kid make solid contact with the golf balls he was swinging at.

Obviously, this young man is not going to be playing a routine game of golf. But anyone who saw him practice would never forget it, wish him the best, and begin to think how he himself could do something for the one he knew needed something badly. Without any doubt, numerous people in real need would receive this in some fashion as the months and years slipped by.

Andrew was absolutely the real father and gentleman, to do what was unusually great; for his young son. It was also obvious to me that Andrew felt extremely proud to watch the improvement in the swing, coming out of that wheelchair.

And so – doesn't this make you want to help others? In some fashion? And not for anything in return, except *thanks*.

THE NUNS OF ISRAEL

There is a very specific reason exactly why I, a Presbyterian, am interested in writing about nuns in

Israel. My wife Franny and our three daughters were longtime visitors in Israel in 1960. I had been invited by Israeli Jewish doctors to operate there in Israel on individuals with head and neck tumors.

Several local Jewish doctors, from Haifa, were driving us north to Haifa one day. They stopped at noon near a huge house and told us that we had been invited there for lunch. We then were told that a large group of nuns lived in this beautiful house and would provide our lunch.

This rather large group of Jewish doctors and the Gaisford family had a superior lunch. We met a number of the nuns who lived there and could not thank them enough for their good cooking and general information about their activities. The doctors with us were very outspoken and told us that they had all been involved in the medical and surgical problems of these nuns and the families that these nuns themselves helped. This was a great experience and was the very beginning of a rather lengthy stay in a wonderful country.

To me, a nun was a female Catholic individual, but I did look up the word in the 4th edition of the American Heritage College Dictionary. Nun:

1.) A woman who belongs to a religious community, living under vows of poverty, chastity and obedience.

2.) The 14th letter of the Hebrew alphabet

The above information from this dictionary made me think about where all of these great nuns had come from and I never really obtained a significant answer. Could some of these nuns be Jews? Were they all Catholic nuns?

My Israeli doctor friends could just not stop talking about the continuous, outstanding great care that these nuns offered to a huge number of people who lived in that country.

This home, where the nuns lived, was quite near to the Sea of Galilee, where the drainage from the southern end became the River Jordan. Incidentally, this Gaisford family walked down to the very beginning of the River Jordan and two of us actually jumped over the River Jordan. I must admit that we initially had to make a jump onto a rock in the middle of this river before we could completely get across.

Jump across the River Jordan some distance south? You had better take a boat!

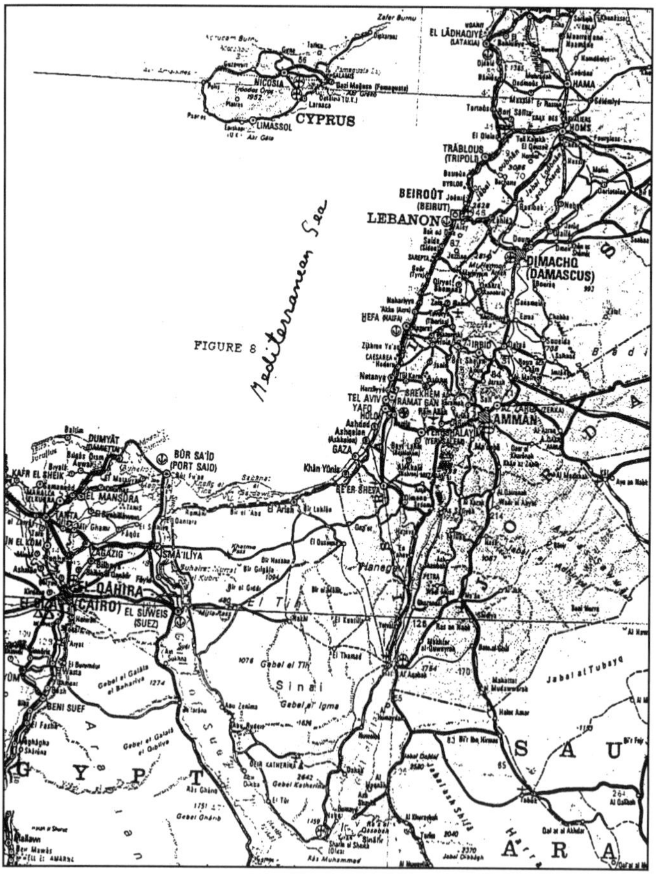

FIGURE 8

Israel is a tiny country but is made up of extremely interesting towns, citics and roads. However, the people who live in Israel could not be more helpful in any possible way.

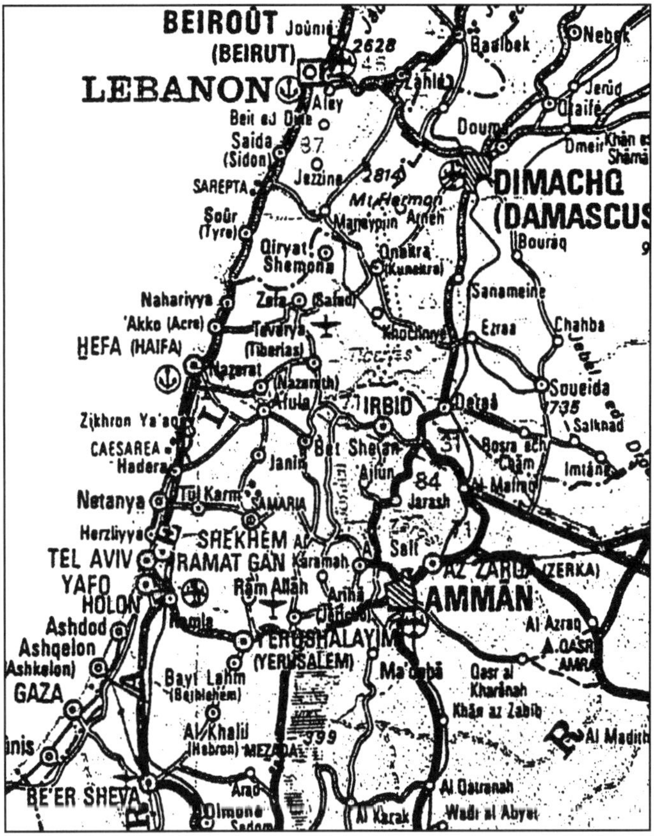

There were many names of cities in this tiny country but one doesn't realize that a tiny country can offer so many world wide and mostly good experiences.

Many countries are adjacent to this tiny Jewish country. Lebanon to the north, Jordan to the west, Egypt to the east and south – and other countries not far away.

Obviously, my association almost 100% of the time was with doctors or hospital personnel. The fact that this large group of nuns was so completely nice in every respect could not be forgotten in any way. I have often thought about the unbelievable things this group of nuns did for so many patients in that little country of Israel. These doctor friends of mine continued to respect the various stories about how these nuns went to extremes to provide help to the patients of my doctor acquaintances. Not acquaintances long – but honest friends immediately.

Probably the most important reason for writing about Israel is not the huge amount of surgery that I undertook there, but how many people the Israeli nuns helped.

A thought that I will promptly follow is this. I was living on the fourth floor of an apartment building in Pittsburgh and on the 6th floor was a friendly Jewish man. He told me one day, when he learned that I had been working in Israel in 1960, that he had gone there to Israel fifteen times. The next time that I see him, I expect to have him tell me absolutely anything he can about the nuns in Israel. Were any of these nuns Jews? I did not tell him that I had been back to Israel about 1980, performing research on a huge burn project for several American companies.

It is difficult just to sit back and think about these Israeli nuns. I sincerely remember what was carried out by these nuns for so many, many individuals of Israel. It was completely obvious that all of these nuns had dedicated their lives just to helping the people who lived in that great little country.

About 1980, I was in the southern part of Israel, near the famous Sea of Galilee, performing research on burn victims, for a well-known American company.

ANTHONY (TONY) BRUNETTE

One of the nicest things that one could discuss is a young man who has been doing things for others. A description of this young man's information and current history should be worth reading. It just so happens that I personally met this boy in 1971, and on October 7, 2008, I talked by phone with his wife.

I walked into the West Penn Hospital Burn/Trauma Unit recently and was greeted by a new nurse. This nurse smiled and introduced himself to me as a former patient of mine. There was time immediately for the two of us to talk, as I was somewhat surprised to have a young man as a burn center nurse. Actually, I didn't even know a male nurse at West Penn Hospital at that period.

This new nurse gave me his name, Anthony (Tony) Brunette, and felt that he had to remind me about the period that he had been my patient. He was sixteen years old at that time. He obviously thought that I could not possibly remember him and his accident, which had occurred in 1971. I think I shocked him somewhat when I related to him how very much I remembered about him. But I just kept quiet and let him talk. What he had done with his life in the aftermath of that accident is remarkable. He reminded me again that he was sixteen at the time of his accident. "I've been busy," he said, "I went to Duquesne University for five years, got a degree in nursing, and early next year, I'm going back for a Master's Degree. I've been teaching young people at Community College but now I've been offered a full time job here in the Burn Center."

I asked Tony if he remembers much about his initial accident and his answers were very interesting.

"I remember everything just like it was yesterday. I was in a car with four of my high school friends when a drunken driver ran into us, killing all four of my friends. I was brought to West Penn Burn/Trauma Unit and you did all of my surgery, as I was really burned."

Tony reminded me of parts of the various operations he was forced to endure. Initially, the most complicated injury problem for both of us was the necessity for performing a total face-lift reconstruction. An interesting part of this facial surgery was the management of the complete loss of all four eyelids – uppers and lowers! This had to be done without delay or both eyes would be lost immediately and permanently.

Tony promptly told me that he could remember one of these operations very clearly. "You said for me to look at my 'new' eyebrows. You had taken strips from the back of my scalp and turned them into eyebrows." This young man was completely correct about the "eyebrow" operation. I had him look at these pieces of skin from his posterior remaining scalp that had relatively normal hair as I would rather promptly begin to reconstruct all four eyelids completely lost to his facial burn and it would be a number of days before he could completely look at anything. These pieces of posterior scalp full thickness skin were then surgically shaped as eyebrows and the surgery of grafting all four eyelids was begun, completed, and the new lower lid was sutured to the new upper lid on the right and the left side. Tony was told that this would be done and that he would be able to see his new eyebrows later, which would then have been placed in the usual eyebrow locations.

The eyelid reconstruction was mandatory, without delay. But the surgery then that was necessary was to reconstruct the entire face – a total face.

Tony then asked me, at an age older than 16, "Did I have a face transplant?" Recently, he had been reading articles about "face transplants," that referred to them as "new" surgical procedures. Tony was informed briefly about the application of only skin used on him and that this was one type of a face transplant; another kind was the reconstruction using skin, muscle, bone and nerves plus blood vessels.

Tony had much more burn damage than a complete third degree (full thickness loss) burn of his face. His hands were third degree totally on the palms and backs and both legs completely from knees to ankles. But – this young man recovered following a number of skin grafts.

This is the time to get right back to Tony. Out of this personal tragedy, he has found a purpose to his life, which enables him to reach out to other patients in a way that very few would ever be able to accomplish. He then, I'm certain, wanted to tell a little more.

"If I hadn't been burned like this," he told me, "I'd never have gone to school to become a nurse and the reason I'm working at West Penn is so that I can help burned people. I think I can do an awful lot for many burned patients. They can see my skin grafted hands and my reconstructed face and ask me any question they want about my experiences as a burned kid."

Tony continues to thank me for being his doctor and for reconstructing various pats of his body, but I don't think he realizes how much I look up to him as an extraordinarily courageous human being who cares so much and so deeply about people.

Who could do more for other people than what Tony has done? Tony has no idea how much he has done for others.

We discussed surgery intensely, but with no relationship to business or money.

MARILYN MCNATT

Marilyn was an absolutely great nurse. She has retired. Following is a rather lengthy description of her years as a working hospital nurse. I knew Marilyn when she worked as a nurse in the usual fashion; later Marilyn worked as a nurse in an unusual fashion.

I asked many questions of Marilyn and she always had superior answers. Were nurses always happy in their work?

All nurses were not happy as nurses so that I put this question to Marilyn. Marilyn promptly stated that too many nurses have kids and they wanted time off to take care of their kids. She felt that money was not the basic interest of the average nurse – but they expected to be paid properly.

Marilyn had a few great remarks, such as, "The nurses in the hospital proper should be paid the most; dealing with families, with doctors and interns – even the administration individuals."

I asked her about hospitals that bring nurses in from other countries, such as the Philippines. Her answers were good ones, that since we in the U.S.A. knew that these nurses had been trained we just put them to work. They were here for one reason – to make money. They are not retrained. She said, "… they go where the pay and working hours are the best they can find."

Marilyn worked at West Penn Hospital for thirty-five years, and for many years before retiring worked in the surgical recovery room. She offered a statement: "I've tried various nursing positions but prefer bedside nursing – hands-on care – so don't put me behind a desk." Another quick answer? "I'm fifty-six years old. I can joke with patients or be serious. Of course, some people can't get along with anybody, so you just do your best, try to help them. I don't see the medical students in this part of surgery but I do work regularly with interns and residents. There is respect between nurses and house staff – but we do handle the occasional young doctor problem."

I then asked Marilyn how nursing in surgical areas had changed during her thirty-five years at West Penn. Her answers were really interesting; patients were treated much better than they were when she began nursing, and many lives now were saved that would not have been years ago.

Marilyn stated that one of the major problems a nurse who worked in the post-surgical area had was that, "the doctor walks in, the patient says he's fine, and as soon as the doctor leaves, we hear the complaints. The doctor never hears a complaint about the food. It's always just fine. But we know there are food and other complaints."

I asked Marilyn about malpractice insurance and she told me that the hospital administration took complete care of those problems and that nurses should not need their own personal insurance.

The most interesting period of talking with Marilyn was about several of her trips outside of Pittsburgh just to help people. This was the most interesting part of the entire meeting with this unusual nurse. At times, several nurses went out of this country just to help in any way that was possible, to help those in nearby countries. Other times doctors and nurses traveled together. Following is a brief remembrance about one trip. "We went to Mexico City twice, last January and August, with my church's blessings. Several doctors and nurses went. Each one of us had to pay his own way, which included airfare and hotels. We set our unit up next to the Mexico City garbage dump – the poorest area in the city. We saw 450 patients in four days on our first trip. We gave out a huge amount of antibiotics that we got from drug companies. And right here, I want to thank you again, Dr. Gaisford, for getting us so many free drugs from Mylan Drug Company. (I was on the Mylan Company Board of Directors at that time.) A lot of these people slept in this garbage dump area, in cardboard rooms or corrugated tin boxes.

"I have been to Mexico several times, the second time, I went with the Assembly of God and Catholic Charities. That time, we saw several hundred patients.

"There's a whole world out there for us to help. Sometimes it tears your heart out, you see terrible things you never saw before. It's just that trying to help people who really need help makes us feel useful. And we will continue to try to help."

It's hard to imagine how much good Marilyn has done for others. Nobody at West Penn Hospital ever knew how Marilyn spent her times away from the hospital. Marilyn had talked with me about the trips, after I had promised never to tell anybody what she had been doing. Now that she has retired and moved, I can talk.

Marilyn moved to South Carolina a number of years ago, having retired from West Penn Hospital. I retired from West Penn several years ago, turned the keys to my two offices in, but was allowed to keep a card to use the parking garage and not pay to park my car.

There is no way that I could ever thank Marilyn enough for not only the help that she and her group gave to the helpless people, but how she actually helped West Penn Hospital doctors, other nurses, and patients within West Penn – a great young lady.

ZENOLA (ZEE) CALLOWAY

One day, January 28, 1999, I was lucky just to have had Zee drop by my office at West Penn Hospital. I asked her to please sit down and we talked. Actually, Zee talked. Zee was retiring in two days, at age 60. She had worked at West Penn for 39 years; her first and only job.

Zee had worked in the operating room areas, mostly in the anesthesia department, but was not a nurse. Zee was a tall, pretty black girl; the first black to have been hired at West Penn Hospital. I just thought it was a proper time just to let Zee – and never knew that her proper first name was Zenola – talk. Following are some of the things brought up by Zee that morning.

"A great servant from the scriptures by the name of James once said 'Life; what is life but a vapor; here for a little while and then it vanishes.' And that really makes you stop and think that is what life is really about. It is here for such a short time and then it vanishes. It is like a vapor, just disappears. So you should make the most out of it. Get the most out of life, because it is not promised and it is not here forever. Here for a little while and then it vanishes."

This first short talk was most unusual, so that I knew that I just wanted Zee to tell me anything.

"My mother brought me up properly. She taught all of us to realize we were somebody. We were poor, we were black, but we didn't feel inferior. I felt proud to work in the operating room. I believe back when I started to work, there was more respect shown. Doctors and nurses cared more about patients than they do now. Our job was completely about patient care. I remember the hospital had a motto then: The Hospital Built on Friendship.

"I am thinking back over 38 years that I worked at West Penn Hospital. Things were so different when I started. It was more like a family unit. Everyone helped each other and had love and respect for all. Dr. Gillespie, Chief of Anesthesia, hired me and at that time, I was the only black. I had so much love and respect for him.

“Our hospital administrator was Mr. James McGuire. He walked throughout the hospital on a regular basis, would hold a door open for you and always asked, ‘How are you?’ It made you feel good that someone that high in office took the time to spend a few minutes with you.

“Then I think of the residency programs we had. These smart young doctors were genuine. We respected them and we could laugh and talk. They could always take the time to listen to us and to the patients.”

It made me realize at this juncture that Zee had done a tremendous amount of good for nurses, interns, residents, administrators and regular doctors. She was first class all the way “helping” in such an unusually quiet, unassuming fashion that many of us never realized how much help we were being offered. I urged her to talk more.

“Maybe more recently, we have lost our thoughts about what we are here for. It should be mandatory for hospital workers to like people. When there is love for people, the job becomes much easier. You will be remembered for the way you treated people as you progress.

“I would love to see the new doctors and all personnel coming into the hospital with the same thought: What can I do to help you? What can I do to help build up this hospital? How can I make patients feel more comfortable and secure? Sometimes everybody isn’t loveable, but there is something good about everybody if you just look and if you take the time to listen for it – it is there. And you doctors just take the time to care about your fellow workers, patients, your hospital, and your doctor friends.

“You new nurses coming in, new medical staff, interns and residents and also administrative people, put yourself into that bed and see how it would feel and how you would like to be treated. Then if you looked at it that way, maybe you will have that compassion and that care to treat that person like you want to be treated. That is the beginning of a great doctor, a great person and that is what you build on. As James said, 'What is life but a vapor, here for a little while and then it vanishes.'"

How would the previous page or two mean anything to someone who might have read them? Possibly it may suggest that the reader just sits back and thinks about how an honest, hard-working black girl lived through the tough times that she experienced. I, personally, looked up to her for all of the things that she had done for so many others. Could there have been any better reason why the operating room got every item it needed or wanted almost instantly from the ones who were just selling equipment? — they were just selling, but they had been associated with Zee for months or years. They respected Zee and because Zee was obviously honest, sincere, and just plain nice, she was one who had done endless things for a variety of people.

SIMON HAFNER

As a general surgical resident in 1948, I assisted in performing a gastrectomy (removal of the stomach) on a Mr. Simon Hafner for cancer of the stomach. There existed a spread of the Stomach cancer had spread to his liver, which means almost certain death in a relatively short time. However, Mr. Hafner did not follow the usual findings and he and I became quite friendly. Simon had come to the United States from Russia at age nine. As time went by, Simon, a Jew, and his wife Florence, a Roman Catholic, became our family friends. Then one day when Simon and I were talking, he was informed that Franny and I were going to Israel. I had been invited to go there to teach head and neck surgery and perform head and neck cancer surgery. Previously, I had been involved in the training of a dentist from Israel and he had arranged for me to work at various Israeli hospitals. When Simon heard about these plans, he hoped that the family, now five (Linda, age 12; Cindy, age 9; and Carolyn, age 7) would have a wonderful time. At that point, all five were not going to go until Simon said, "I'm paying for everything," and he did by giving me $25,000. Twenty-five thousand dollars is a lot of money today, but in 1961, it was a lot of money. In addition, Simon gave me considerably more money to use in Israel in any way I could use it to improve medical care for the people of Israel ($75,000).

After a stop or two we arrived in Tel Aviv and were met by our Israeli friends. While touring around a new country was extremely enlightening, the medical aspect of the visit was even more educational. I was pleasantly surprised to realize very quickly the high caliber of medicine and surgery that was practiced throughout Israel. My initial introduction to a hospital there was the Hadassah University in Tel Aviv. The plastic surgeon there invited me to work with him, which operation was not too unlike the same type of procedure in Pittsburgh. The noticeable difference began with the very careful technique of actually collecting the water running from the spigots as we scrubbed our hands before operating. It was quite obvious that water was at a premium. In addition, this very modern institution had an excessive supply of surgical equipment. I remembered that, as the days passed, the Hadassah women in the United States were extremely active and had overdone themselves in working so hard for this one university hospital. The other hospitals I visited and became quite well acquainted with were really in need of equipment and outside assistance.

It did not take but a few telephone calls and several hours to become acquainted with a number of doctors there in Israel. Many of my new doctor friends were from Haifa, in the northern section of Israel, but not very far from Tel Aviv.

This nice group of physicians from Haifa invited me to go with them to Haifa and give some talks on my knowledge about head and neck tumors. One day, these doctors picked my entire family up and drove us to Haifa, where we were placed in a hotel near where these doctors worked – Ram Bam Hospital. We remained in Haifa for several days to a week.

Ram Bam Hospital was an extremely well organized and efficient institution. While in that area, I began to see many head and neck tumor cases and began operating as the operating surgeon. One particular case, a very difficult parotidectomy and radical neck dissection, brought back thoughts of my work with the Japanese surgeon at the Imperial University Hospital in Japan. Neither my anesthetist nor scrub nurses could speak English at the Ram Bam Hospital, but operating room personnel in almost every country probably think alike – there were no problems for me in Israel.

A considerable amount of Simon's money was used to improve the equipment deficits at Ram Bam Hospital. In addition to the equipment situation, I established a foundation in the name of Simon Hafner at Ram Bam Hospital, there in Haifa. Some of the Hafner money was used to purchase necessary materials in other Israeli hospitals.

Possibly my description of Israeli hospital problems, exclusive of Hadasah University, to my many Pittsburgh Jewish lady friends may have contributed to their spreading their generous gifts to other Israeli hospitals. Several doctors associated with the Haifa Hospital did remarkable things. It was, of course, not possible to perform surgery on the large number of head and neck tumor problems that were presented to me. I would examine these patients with their physicians and suggest how they could be adequately and properly managed. As mentioned, I operated on selected patients. An unforgettable follow up occurred. Over the year following our return home, these hard-working doctors kept me apprised about every patient we had seen together and had outlined care for. Little did I realize that in 1990, 29 years later, I would be back in Israel operating again. This trip took me to Beer Sheva, sandwiched between the Gaza Strip and the West Bank, in the Negev Desert.

A number of years later, Simon died and left me $750,000 to use at West Penn Hospital at my discretion. Part of that was used to set up the first outpatient surgical department at West Penn, named in memory of Florence and Simon Hafner. When a more modern department was constructed and the heavy bronze plaque with Florence and Simon Hafner's name was taken down, that bronze plaque was delivered to me, and it resides in my office beside my desk in the Mellon Pavilion today!

Simon and Florence Hafner could never have known how much they did for so many people in the United States and in Israel, for people they had never met and had not known about. One word about Florence. This real lady had grown up a Roman Catholic, and then she married Simon, a Jew. One night at dinner at the Jewish Westmoreland Country Club in Pittsburgh, Florence leaned over to me and said, "You know, I'm a better Jew than Simon, my husband, and you are his best friend, and not a Jew."

11 || PEOPLE (BUSINESS & GOLF)

A Poem About
Golfers Who Play on Sunday Mornings

The Lord watcheth over me, I will not score well.

He maketh balls to lie down in deep rough.

He leadeth shots into still waters.

He restoreth my slice.

He leadeth me down the wrong cart path confused for His name's sake.

Yea, though I drive past the alley of the shadow of doom, I will fear many pitfalls for thou art against me.

Thou preparest a fast green before me in the presence of my foursome.

Thou anointest my brow with sweat.

My ball runneth over the cup.

Surely birdies and pars shall elude me all the days of my life;

Till I dwell in the house of the Lord on Sunday mornings.

– author unknown

PEOPLE

There always have been and always will be people who work, make money by working, and have to work to pay their bills.

But, there is currently a very interesting game – golf – that not only is played by superior players but those who just play. The game frequently is involved with business or is just a way to spend some time. Business quite often is mixed with golf – for very different reasons.

The following will create some questions.

SAM PARKS

Surgery, golf, and business can be combined in a variety of ways. Following is a discussion as to how these three extremely important groups can intermix at times. This author has been involved in a variety of ways.

Sam Parks was the head professional at the South Hills Country Club, near downtown Pittsburgh, Pennsylvania, when he won the National Open at the Oakmont Country Club in 1932.

Sam proved without any doubt that real practice, whether it be golf, surgery, or whatever would be absolutely helpful for that individual.

Sam ended his golfing career in 1970, took a job with U.S. Steel and moved to Florida. His family members were my patients before they moved. In 1985, I played my last game of golf with Sam, in Florida. He died in 1998.

ED FURGOL

Ed Furgol was an unusual individual. He will always be remembered as the great golfer with the "withered" left arm, the result of an accident. Ed won the National Open in 1954 at Baltimore Golf Club in Springfield, New Jersey. His left elbow was fixed at a 45-degree angle and could not even be physically flexed or extended but a small fraction. Ed came to Pittsburgh as head professional of the Westmoreland Country Club after his National Open win, and the only notable win he had around Pittsburgh was the West Penn Open in 1965.

Later, Ed came to me as a patient. He wanted me to fix his left elbow so that it would be normal, working like his good right arm. All this was after he had won the National Open with his bad left arm. He was too big for me to toss out of the office after his dumb request – but we did play a lot of golf together.

Playing with Ed with his peculiar golf swing due to his peculiar left arm and how he had to train a variety of muscles to perform differently from the way they were usually designed, gave me a lot to think about.

I performed a lot of hand surgery over the years and could not help but discuss Ed's physical arm problems and how he was such a great golfer even with his severe physical deformity with some of my patients who voiced a variety of complaints.

BOBBY CRUICKSHANK

Bobby Cruickshank was without a doubt one of the best-known professional golfers of his time. Bobby never won the National Open, but almost. He was an unusual individual and had come to the United States from Carnousti, Scotland, along with Tommy Armour and many other golf professionals.

Bobby played many professional golf tournaments before becoming the head professional at the

Chartiers Country Club in Pittsburgh. He stayed there until his death.

I knew a lot about him being a great golfer long before we met. While I had followed him at various Pittsburgh professional tournaments, we had not met until he was referred to me as a surgical patient.

Bobby was almost a great winner, having lost in an 18-hole playoff against Bobby Jones at the Merion Golf Club in Philadelphia in 1932 for the National Open title.

Possibly the best known story about him was the article in the January 1979 issue of *Golf Magazine*, written by Al Watrous, another superb golfer. Incidentally, Al Watrous's son and I know each other through memberships in the American Seniors Golf Association. A lot can be learned by reading the following article about how never giving up refers not only to golf but to many, many situations. This golf article is well worth reading.

He was nine down with 12 holes to play, but Wee Bobby Cruickshank never gave up. Here's the full story of the most spectacular come-from-behind victory in PGA Championship history, told by the man who was beaten. (*Golf Magazine* 01/79)

Al Waltrous told his story in this detailed multiple page letter about his loss to Bobby – Al was 80 years old then, in 1979. I'm rewriting this story in 2009.

In 1965, I saw Bobby as a patient. Bobby always played with his hat pulled down over his forehead, especially low on the right, and he never removed that hat regardless of where he was. When the hat was removed, it was very obvious why he always wore it – an extremely large skin tumor, about 10 square inches in size, was quite noticeable. After an examination, it was obvious to me that surgery was definitely indicated – a somewhat radical excision of this tumor and reconstruction. A biopsy revealed the growth to be malignant. Bobby was not a teetotaler, but it was elected to perform this surgery under local anesthesia for several reasons. Local anesthesia would be safer and Bobby seemed to be comfortable with this approach to his problem. And then we immediately began talking golf.

On the day of the scheduled surgery, Bobby was admitted to Allegheny General Hospital, given his preoperative medicine and taken to the operating room. I knew it would be a long operation and expected it to be a problem. However, it turned out to be an extremely interesting three-hour operation, as Bobby never stopped talking. I don't think he ever felt a thing.

As I began to inject Bobby with a local anesthetic, I asked him if the article I had read involving Al Watrous and himself was true – that Bobby was nine down with twelve to play and he beat Watrous?

Bobby almost shouted and I thought he might even just try to sit up on the operating table to discuss this question. He answered promptly, "..that was 1932, the PGA, I'm playing like a toad and Al Watrous is killing me…" Well, it was an interesting operation and conversation. Bobby got really excited and started to talk about that day. He started by describing the first hole, and remembered every shot each one had hit, how he lost many holes and then began to win hole after hole after being far behind. And you know how it ended – Bobby won. He evened the 36-hole match on the 36th hole and won the match on the 40th hole – four extra holes.

The telling, remembering, and replaying of that match was a real education for us in the operating room. No one seemed to be overly concerned about the surgery and everything did turn out well. Just about the time Bobby sank his last putt on the 40th hole, the rather large skin graft was completely sewed into place in the large defect in scalp and forehead. (I can't remember where I obtained the graft.)

But Bobby never stopped wearing that pulled-down golf hat!

Bobby recovered with no complications and we became golfing friends. Because Bobby was a good friend of Willie McKay at Longue Vue, both having come here from Scotland, occasionally we would play together at the Longue Vue Club. However, most of our golf together was played at Fox Chapel Golf Club.

One day in 1969, Carolyn, the youngest of our three daughters, played golf with Bobby, Fox Chapel professional Bill Downing and me. Carolyn was riding with Bobby in a cart and I heard her ask Bobby if he could tell or show her how to get out of sand bunkers because she felt inept about the technique. Bobby displayed a very professional answer. He did not answer Carolyn by describing the way to solve that problem and did not offer to show her what to do. He did not answer her in the way many amateurs would answer but gave her an excellent answer, "Carolyn, Mr. Downing is your Fox Chapel Club teaching professional. He is going to be available for help on a regular basis. It is my opinion that he is extremely capable of helping you with this sand problem. So, to make it easy on you and get your problem solved, go see Mr. Downing. It will be convenient, you will be shown how to handle this problem, and it's the smartest thing to do."

I agreed with Bobby. Carolyn went on to win the club championship at a later date.

UNKNOWN GOLF PROFESSIONAL FROM WEST VIRGINIA

All golf games and all surgical operations do not always terminate in good results. This situation fits that statement.

There is no way that I could ever come up with this particular golf professional's name – but he will never be forgotten. He was a patient, a young man, and was referred to me for surgery following the amputation of his right arm. Obviously, nothing could be done surgically to replace such a loss, but I did operate on him. And this professional was professional in every way. He gave me a gift and not because he wasn't charged for my surgery. The gift? – his favorite tee. This tee was a combined long and short tee, connected by an eight-inch, chain, all of sterling silver. He stated with a wry smile, "I'm not going to need my favorite tees anymore." I have never used these tees – never will – but they have a permanent home in my golf bag. I have given my golf bag and clubs away, but not these tees.

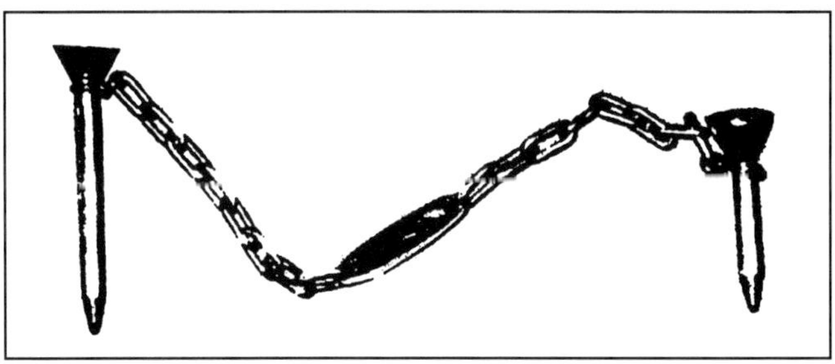

STERLING SILVER GOLF TEES

How I wish I could remember the name of this young golf professional. I thought of him every time I felt this gift of tees when I reached into a certain pocket in my golf bag. And the first time this year that I have been outside to hit golf balls – March 2009 – I made an effort to get all those ancient 2008 golf balls out of my bag, and I felt this sterling silver pair of golf tees.

TOM WATSON

Tom Watson is a real gentleman. Tom was from Kansas City, went to Stanford University, and knew our next-door neighbors, the Michaels, who were also from Kansas City. In addition, their son, Mike had graduated from Stanford. The National Open was being held at Oakmont that year, 1983, and Tom, his wife Linda, and the Gaisfords had dinner out on the Michaels's patio the evening before the four-day tournament.

Tom did not drink any alcohol, but later that evening, after we had left, while opening a bottle of Coca-Cola, he cut the front flat side of his right index finger. Mike promptly brought Tom over to our house to obtain my super expert medical help. He looked like a little kid, sitting on the couch in the library with his right hand sticking up in the air – the National Open to begin the next morning and he with a cut finger.

The injury did not demand stitches, but was adequately, firmly approximated side to side. And Tom showed unusual acceptance of this unfortunate, small but quite bothersome injury. He made me promise that no one should be told about his injury. He did not want to use his hand laceration as an excuse for whatever might happen during the following four days.

And what did happen? On Sunday, the fourth and last day of the National Open, Tom was doing extremely well. He was playing with Larry Nelson and was in position on the last of the 72-hole tournament to tie Nelson and cause a play-off. Larry was down with a birdie 3 and Tom had to chip in from just off the putting surface to tie. He missed, and was, of course, second.

Oakmont hosted the National Open in 1996. Tom did not come close to winning, but we did have a short visit at Franco's restaurant. Soon after that, he sent me an autographed photograph, which was much appreciated.

One additional comment about Tom. He has won the British Open Golf Tournament five times. No one else has even come close to that number of wins. And in 2008, Tom was playing in the senior tour.

There are many golf professionals with whom I have had contact over the years. But enough talk about golf professionals, this is sufficient. That is, except for a few stories about professionals and nonprofessionals – in situations involving golf-surgery-business. *Many* times, this trio of golf-surgery-business gets tangled—at times, in a surreptitious fashion.

LEON OLIVER
Bartender and Golf Professional

RICHARD HORNBERGER, MD
Chest Surgeon

Not all great players are National Open Champions and not all surgeons are professors of surgery. But they can be great in various ways.

Leon Oliver was a bartender when I met him in the Gasparilla Inn at Boca Grande, Florida. Leon is from the state of Maine where, during the summer seasons, he is head golf professional at the Wawenock Country Club at Walpole, Maine. I had played in a January golf tournament at Gasparilla, became friends with Leon, and played a lot of golf with him, including the day that he set a new course record of 63, eight under par. And then in 2006, Leon had become the maitre d' in the dining area at the Gasparilla Inn.

Approximately twenty years ago, an invitation was extended to me to become a member of the Gasparilla "48" Club. I accepted the invitation. No one, however, has figured out how the "48" Club name originated. The Gasparilla Inn and Cottages compound is on Gasparilla Island at Boca Grande, Florida. The "48" Club is an old, old club made up of senior golfers. This low-key hotel complex is just a comfortable place to spend a short vacation.

The golf facilities are more than acceptable, the golf course itself always in perfect condition, and more than enough for me from those too-far-back tees. It has been my good fortune to have met and become associated with numerous interesting and well-known people. Titles are dropped and no one has ever addressed me as "Dr. Gaisford." One day, while playing with bartender, Leon Oliver, and two new acquaintances, Leon poked me, as we were putting out on the 13th green. He pointed to a house across the inlet, possibly a hundred yards away, to tell me that my one playing partner lived there – Admiral Chester Nimitz. What had I been calling Admiral Nimitz up to that point? I think it was "Chete."

Leon knew that I had a M*A*S*H unit in the Pacific in World War II and mentioned one day that a member of this club, a Dr. Richard Hornberger, had such a unit in the Korean War and was the individual who arranged for the development of the M*A*S*H television series. Leon had mentioned to him that I had such a unit in 1945. I just had to speak with Dr. Hornberger. So I called him on the telephone after Leon had given me his telephone number and I had returned to Pittsburgh. We had a nice visit and I casually mentioned to him that I thought my next-door neighbor might have been his commanding officer in Korea. Dr. Hornberger said he didn't think that would be possible, but when I told him that my next-door neighbor was General Matthew B. Ridgway, he dropped the telephone.

We thoroughly discussed our M*A*S*H unit experience, and I told Dr. Hornberger that the M*A*S*H television episodes were the only TV shows I watched. He then promised to arrange for me to meet "Hawkeye" – Alan Alda.

Arrangements were made to play golf with Dr. Hornberger and my bartender golf professional, Leon Oliver. On June 15, 1996 at 7:00 AM, I flew to New York, changed planes and reached Portland at 11:00 AM. A rental car got me really lost about five times trying to find Leon's little nine-hole golf course. The town of Walpole is 60 miles north of Portland, but Leon's club was not near any town or house. However, I did get a free sandwich and had a truly memorable day, playing golf with Dr. Hornberger, discussing our past common experiences, and just spending the day with down-to-earth people. Leon, being the head professional at this club, Wawenock Country Club, also was "head" of everything else. While one young woman made lunches, another ran the so-called golf shop. There was a "driving range" near the first tee. Buckets of balls could be hit, but those balls were not made in this decade, had never been cleaned, and flew reluctantly. After our golf game (and I rode in a rather balky car with Dr. Hornberger), I said goodbye to Dr. Hornberger and then went out into a soggy, bug-infested, swampy driving range to help Leon (the "head" professional) attempt to retrieve all those rocks that had been knocked off a so-called teeing area. I wouldn't give anything for my Maine – more accurately "main" experience.

That was my only meeting with Dr. Hornberger, and on November 9, 1997, his death notice appeared in the *Pittsburgh Post-Gazette.*

PITTSBURGH POST GAZETTE
SUNDAY, NOVEMBER 9, 1997

OBITUARIES

H. Richard Hornberger, 73, a surgeon whose novel inspired the television series "M*A*S*H," Tues-day in Portland, Maine. The TV show and the hit movie were based on the novel of the same name that Dr. Hornberger, a thoracic surgeon who lived in Bremen, wrote after serving with a Mobile Army Surgi-cal Hospital during the Korean War. He wrote two sequels to the book and maintained an active surgical practice in Waterville, Maine, until his retirement in 1988.

DR. HORNBERGER WAS A UNIQUE, SMALL TOWN SURGEON. WE DEVELOPED A SINCERE FRIENDSHIP AS WE COMPLETELY UNDERSOOD OUR FORMERLY INDESCRIBABLE M*A*S*H UNIT PROBLEMS AND EXPERIENCES. THERE WOULD HAVE BEEN NO REAL OPPORTUNITY FOR ME TO HAVE MET THIS FINE, INTERESTING MAN HAD I NOT GOTTEN TO KNOW A CERTAIN BARTENDER—LEON OLIVER.

The death notice of a Mr. Henry Cannon was on the same page with Dr. Hornberger. He was the husband of the famous movie star and stage star, Minnie Pearl. Many years ago, we had become well acquainted with Minnie Pearl (a personal friend through surgery and not golf) of the Grand Ole Opry fame, in Nashville, Tennessee. We had a daughter at Vanderbilt University.

Some years ago, Franny and I splurged and flew down for an extra week at Gasparilla. Since it was spring break for many schools, our daughter, Cindy, her husband, Jack, and his mother, along with Cindy's and Jack's two pretty, young daughters, Collyer and Carrie, made up our group. There were kids everywhere.

Collyer and Carrie hooked up with two other young ones, began playing a lot of ping-pong with them, and they all became friends. A surprise – the two new "kids" belonged to George W. Bush (before he became president). At that time, Mr. George W. Bush was working with his Texas Rangers ball team about 30 miles from Gasparilla. Unfortunately, we never had the opportunity to meet the children's parents, but the senior past president and wife, Barbara, were there – babysitters.

Golf is a favorite for former President George H. W. Bush. One day when we and the Klees were there together, the golf course was somewhat busy. Mr. Bush was playing and I would have given anything to have been invited to play with him. Our several foursomes were playing rather close together, and the somewhat nasty rain made the decision for us to hang it up.

We initially met and talked with Mr. Bush outside the pro shop. Our daughter, Cindy Klee, a very adequate golfer, is not a shy young lady. She struck up a conversation with President Bush and then asked him if she could take his picture. President Bush's answer? "Sure, Cindy, if you'll get in the picture with me." Cindy later said, "And he really squeezed me!"

This day certainly was a wet one. Mr. Bush looked like, was, and is, a regular guy. Here he was, with wet, straggly hair, but that didn't bother him a bit. And the Bushes were comfortable normal people – standing in line with the rest of us to pick up lunch, talking with numerous well-wishers, just being a wonderful couple.

Mrs. Barbara Bush was such a down-to-earth regular individual; she became an unbelievably popular person.

A surgical meeting in Dallas some years ago led to an extraordinary golf experience. A surgical friend living in Dallas invited me to Preston Trail Golf Links for lunch and golf. My golf partner was Byron Nelson, a shocking surprise to me. But lunch was in some respects more shocking. I sat between Byron and Buddy Dial. Buddy, at one time, was a Pittsburgh Steeler and a great player. At this particular time, he was quite crippled from football injuries, but a most interesting individual. I had heard his name and read athletic reports about him, but this was our first meeting.

As if I hadn't been surprised enough, Byron and Buddy started to laugh, just as a helicopter was landing extremely close to the veranda and our table. All Byron said was, "He's late again" – and a rather young, nicely dressed man stepped up and sat down at the table with us. Byron introduced me to him, and I still haven't completely recovered. The "young man" was Lamar Hunt, one of the richest men in the country. Later, as I read in the paper, he and other members of his family managed to establish close links to the United States government when they tried to corner the silver market – which cost the Hunt group millions. I learned that Lamar Hunt and Byron played a lot of golf together – and money became a huge help for Byron.

Having shared Byron's locker with him, I helped myself to an old, beat-up ball that in some way got into his locker. Writing to him later, I mentioned that I had stolen that ball.

After I returned home from this surgery-golf trip, I learned a lot about Byron. He stopped playing professional golf tournaments rather promptly after winning eight tournaments in a row, but he then appeared to have a quite large amount of money. Could there have been any connection in business with the Hunt family?

Speaking of interesting golf stories, here is one never to be forgotten. Several years ago, there was an article in the *Readers' Digest* magazine about a blind lawyer. The "blind lawyer," Bob Ahlmon, happened to have been a classmate of mine at the University of Pennsylvania, 1934-1938, and I had a lot in common with Bob. He had been injured at age eight, falling off a freight car on which he should not have been playing, becoming completely and permanently blinded.

All Bob's classes were such that books in Braille were not always available. Countless times, I would read to Bob from books in the classes we shared. I really spent hours reading my (our) college books to Bob.

What does all this have to do with golf? It fits perfectly. Wouldn't it be much easier for a blind person to listen to the television or be plugged into a computer than to have a book read to him? But practice and play golf? These blind golfers were not quitters in any way.

Some years ago, the National Blind Golfers tournament was held at the Fox Chapel Golf Club, and I was local chairman of the event. I scanned the entry list and found Bob's name. Obviously, we renewed our friendship and while Bob did not win the tournament, he played unbelievably well.

On the last night of the tournament, my wife and I had Bob and his wife over for dinner at Fox Chapel. I couldn't help but ask him how he always got A's in all his subjects and I got C's. His answer? "All I had to do was reach in my pocket and read off notes in Braille."

There was no end to meeting golfers who make the meeting interesting. (Haven't you ever met an avid golfer who could beat you with his story after you thought you were a winner? Of course!)

It is with considerable pleasure through countless remembrances that this section on golf professionals is undertaken. This small group of real professionals included friends, patients, short-term acquaintances – no matter. These men were all extremely talented in one way or another, and I was just a very lucky individual to have become associated with them in some fashion.

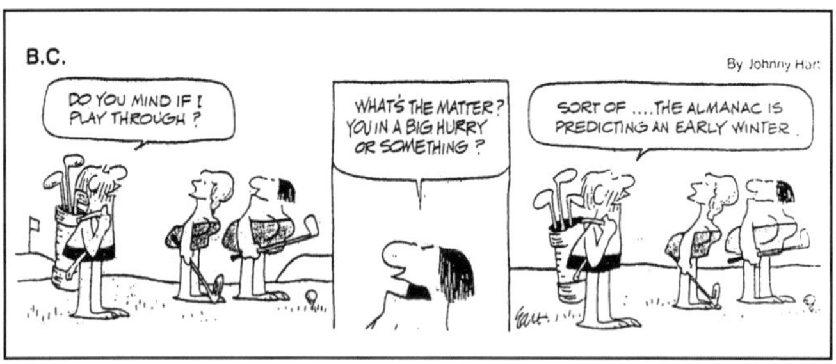
B.C.
By Johnny Hart
DO YOU MIND IF I PLAY THROUGH ?
WHAT'S THE MATTER? YOU IN A BIG HURRY OR SOMETHING ?
SORT OF ....THE ALMANAC IS PREDICTING AN EARLY WINTER .

The above cartoon represents a never-ending joke among lots of men when it comes to golf played by numerous females. This particular joke struck me as a good one – with a wife and three daughters – all of whom have played a lot of golf. All have looked at this joke on multiple occasions; who would have shown it to them? All of this work at a golf club is work – plus lots of fun.

It's becoming more and more difficult not to bring golf into the picture, so that more is on the way, while there will be talk involving golf and surgery.

Surgeons perform various types of surgery and as a qualified reconstructive surgeon this surgeon was presented with the unusual request one day for surgery. The patient was a 45-year-old, very nice looking lady, who had an unusual request. She wanted her left breast reduced markedly in size, for a special reason: "My breasts are very large and the left breast really gets in my way when I swing my golf club back to the right."

Examination of this golfing female did reveal very large breasts; but reduce one of the two in size? She was extremely sincere in her request, but I convinced her that a better solution would be to reduce the size of both breasts, which would promptly make her more comfortable. Also, she probably would score better on the golf course.

A bilateral operation was performed and while it would appear to the operating surgeon, who was also interested in golf, that this young women's golf score would be improved, no scorecards were ever produced for evaluation.

Numerous things happen on golf courses, and all are not good. One of the worst neck injuries was the result of a game of golf and a golf club was brought to me one afternoon. This teen-aged boy had knocked his ball around in some trees on a side hill and when he attempted to free it with an eight iron, the head of the club struck a tree, breaking the club in half. This boy then stumbled, fell face forward against the hill, falling against the open metal shaft, which went into his neck, with that end protruding from the opposite side of his neck.

The golf professional and his staff at that golf club performed in an outstanding safe fashion. Instead of pulling that metal shaft out of the neck, from either the right or left side, that boy was immediately brought to me at West Penn Hospital.

I had never seen such an accident and promptly operated on this boy, opening his neck with an incision, which extended from one earlobe to the other, turning wide skin and muscle flaps up and down. I thought that this metal tube could have damaged one of the large blood vessels in the neck, and exposing the path of this golf club shaft would permit me to manage any injury in a safe fashion.

And what was found? Not one blood vessel or important nerve was injured. The metal shaft was removed without any difficulty whatsoever since it had been completely surgically exposed, and the neck incision was repaired.

The golf professional had made the absolutely correct decision not to pull that golf club shaft out. Had an artery or vein of any size been injured, that golf club shaft may have been holding pressure against it, preventing bleeding, and extracting the shaft could have removed temporary pressure, then causing the death of that boy from blood loss.

Are some golf course medical or surgical experiences reasonable to discuss? I think so, but this particular one turned out to be somewhat different. It just happened that the golfer/patient happened to be an internationally known individual, the Ambassador of the United States of America, on vacation from Paris, France. He was Walter J. P. Curley.

This was 1976 and it was customary at the Fox Chapel Golf Club that, after completion of the first nine holes of golf, a stop could, and usually would, be made at the sandwich shop near the tenth tee. I took advantage of what I thought would be my opportunity to grab a sandwich quickly, drink a cup of black coffee, tee up a golf ball and hit a perfect drive, and then move to allow the following group at least to take advantage of the two bathrooms.

However, various strange things can occur on a golf course, and this particular problem was really not too strange for a doctor. A very nice appearing young man, obviously informed by those who had been playing golf with him that I was a doctor who was active in head and neck surgery, got up from the small table where he was sitting and introduced himself.

"I'm Walter Curley. I fell yesterday and I'm having difficulty seeing clearly. My playing partners have told me that you know face problems, and I wonder if you would just take a minute and look at what seems to me to possibly be a crack in my cheek bone."

It took but a minute to discover upon the examination of Walter Curley's face that he had a rather severe fracture of his right upper jaw and that his right eye was involved. Obviously, to me, the floor of his right orbit – the bone that the right eye rests on – was broken, and surgery certainly was indicated.

And then I realized just who Walter Curley was – our ambassador to France. The name, Curley, was well known to me and to the Fox Chapel Golf Club and its members; I had to make a prompt decision regarding his facial injury.

I asked Mr. Curley where he lived and he told me he had an apartment in New York City and that he had planned on returning to New York in a day or two. When I asked him his address in New York, it just happened that his apartment was within a city block of where Dr. John Converse lived. Dr. Converse, a personal friend of mine for years, was Professor of Reconstructive Surgery at New York University and the accepted leader in the United States on facial bone reconstruction.

Mr. Curley and I decided that I would attempt to contact Dr. Converse that day and ask that he see Mr. Curley promptly. That afternoon I made a call to John Converse, and he stated that he would be available to see his patient the following day if the patient could return to New York promptly. Dr. Converse and I both thought that prompt surgery was indicated.

Walter Curley was seen the following day by Dr. Converse with surgery being planned for the next morning. Things went as planned. Surgery was performed, and the result was perfect. The fact that the result was perfect was proven because the use of the damaged eye area allowed perfect vision to be restored.

Back to golf. Although it was not mentioned previously, Walter Curley's home was in Fox Chapel. He was born at his home on Fairway Lane, the entrance to which is approximately 90 yards from the entrance to the Fox Chapel Golf Club.

Discussion regarding the name Curley is not quite over. A golf tournament that has been extremely popular at the Fox Chapel Golf club for many years is the Curley Cup Tournament. The tournament had been established many years ago, involving just members of the Fox Chapel Golf Club and partners in the event being a male and a female. What happened one year? My youngest daughter, Carolyn, and I won it. This was in 1990.

EMBASSY OF THE UNITED STATES OF AMERICA
PARIS

THE AMBASSADOR

September 6, 1990

Dear Mrs. Morris and Dr. Gaisford:

I am late in congratulating you both on winning The Curley Cup Tournament Low Net in 1990. I salute you for your excellent play, and I want you to know how pleased we are that you are participants in this competition which was established so many years ago by my parents for low-handicap golfers.

Warmest wishes and congratulations.

Yours sincerely,

Walter J.P. Curley

Mrs. Carolyn Morris
1026 Heberton Street
Pittsburgh, Pennsylvania

Dr. John Gaisford
910 West Waldheim Road
Pittsburgh, Pennsylvania

John – do you remember 'attending' to my blow-out fracture (skate-board!) years ago? I just had another operation (cataract / Dr. Dodick) recently that worked well.
Best wishes.
Walter

A LETTER TO ME FROM AMBASSADOR WALTER CURLEY.

John C. Gaisford, M.D.

Mellon Pavilion Suite 340
4815 Liberty Avenue
Pittsburgh, PA 15224

Telephone
(412) 681-5266

October 2, 1990

The Honorable Walter J. P. Curley
American Ambassador
Paris
Embassy of the United States of America
2 Avenue Gabriel
75382 Paris Cedex 08, France

My Dear Mr. Ambassador:

Thank you so much for your nice letter regarding the Curley Cup Tournament. I'm sure your parents would never have imagined that this Tournament would be the most popular of matches among the Pittsburgh area clubs.

The Mrs. Morris, who was my partner, just happens to be my youngest daughter -- a former Fox Chapel Club Champion.

I certainly do remember the blow-out fracture you suffered. Am I correct in remembering that you fell off Elsie Hillman's skate board? I'm glad your recent eye procedure went well.

Thanks again, and with kindest personal regards, I am

Sincerely yours,

Jack Gaisford

John C. Gaisford, M.D.

A LETTER TO AMBASSADOR CURLEY FROM ME.

The Laurel Valley Country Club in Ligonier, Pennsylvania, is one of the finest golf courses and clubs in the United States. Numerous groups arrange with this club to have their golf outings there, and one beautiful June day in 1995, the Pittsburgh law firm Reed Smith met there for lunch, golf, cocktails and dinner. There is a lot of money for a golf club for this type of an outing.

Curt Siegel was the golf professional at Laurel Valley and in addition to performing the routine work done by the professional of an active golf club, he was also a professional at golf club tricks.

As the several dozen Reed Smith lawyers were waiting outside the dining room at the Arnold Palmer Pavilion, having a glass of water or something and looking down over the edge of this stone porch, Curt Siegel began performing his golf tricks. Curt had informed everyone that they might be interested in what he had to offer, and many among that group of lawyers knew that Curt was an excellent performer, having previously seen some of what he had to offer.

This particular evening was a little different when it came to his showing off a personal, new trick. Curt had everyone's attention when he showed off a six-and-a-half foot long driver and swung it back and forth, showing that it was so limber that it appeared similar to one whipping a length of rather heavy wire the diameter of a golf club. Curt had the head of a golf club driver attached to the end of this wire-like shaft and was hitting balls with this club in an unbelievably professional fashion.

Suddenly Curt looked up and asked if anyone had a wristwatch that he could use. He would place the watch on the ground, face up, put a golf ball on it and drive that ball off the watch. He stated that he knew what he was doing in a safe fashion.

Curt glanced up and caught my eye, as he and I had known each other for years. I was at this golf and dinner with these lawyers, even though I was not in their legal business. I tossed Curt my wristwatch, he placed it on the ground with the face up, placed a golf ball on it, and then took a couple of practice swings. He then stepped up to my watch with the golf ball on it, and as several dozen lawyers watched, Curt took this unbelievably wide, bending swing at that ball only to have the head of his golf club hit golf ball, my watch and dirt, with glass, metal and golf ball flying somewhere northwest.

Everyone watching this golf trick by the head professional at Laurel Valley groaned and asked for another drink. Several looked at me, a couple told me to make Curt get me another watch, and I probably just slithered over to the pro shop.

What this group of lawyers didn't know was that I had played a lot of golf with Curt, at Laurel Valley and Fox Chapel Golf Club, and that my good personal wristwatch was at the club house and Curt had arranged this entire golf trick earlier. He had given me a cheap wristwatch earlier in the day to toss down to him when he asked if anyone had a wristwatch to loan him so that he could show how great a golfer he was.

Later that evening, Curt gave it away, that it was a prearranged golf trick. I'm sure that Curt didn't want those lawyers to think that he had just messed up that trick for fear he might not be asked to perform at another party. It was a good dinner party!

And isn't the name of this section Golf-Medicine-Business? And isn't the following picture of a golf ball invitation sent by Roy McKnight, somewhat interesting? This is really good golf-medicine-business.

Roy McKnight was CEO of Mylan laboratories, Inc. and had made that company the leader of generic drug companies in the United States.

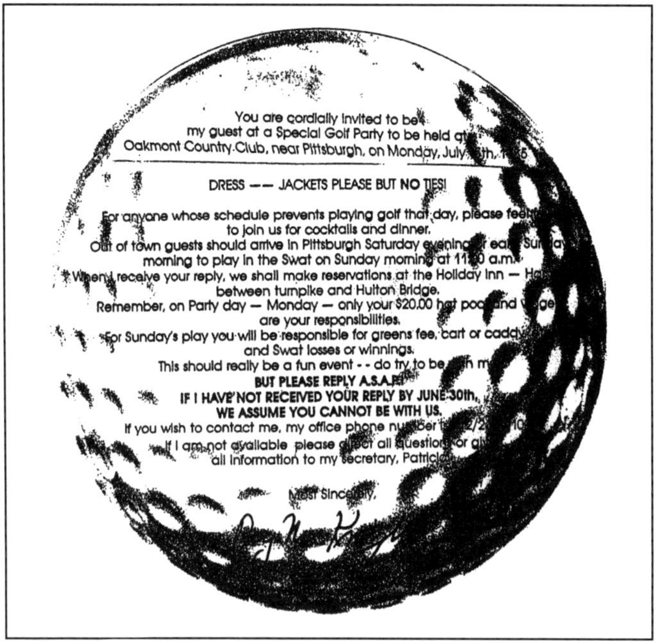

You are cordially invited to be
my guest at a Special Golf Party to be held at
Oakmont Country Club, near Pittsburgh, on Monday, July [illegible]th, [illegible]

DRESS — — JACKETS PLEASE BUT NO TIES!

For anyone whose schedule prevents playing golf that day, please feel [illegible]
to join us for cocktails and dinner.
Out of town guests should arrive in Pittsburgh Saturday evening or early Sunday
morning to play in the Swat on Sunday morning at 11:[illegible]0 a.m.
When I receive your reply, we shall make reservations at the Holiday Inn — Ha[illegible]
between turnpike and Hulton Bridge.
Remember, on Party day — Monday — only your $20.00 hat pool and w[illegible]ge[illegible]
are your responsibilities.
For Sunday's play you will be responsible for greens fee, cart or caddy [illegible]
and Swat losses or winnings.
This should really be a fun event - - do try to be with m[illegible]
BUT PLEASE REPLY A.S.A.P.!
IF I HAVE NOT RECEIVED YOUR REPLY BY JUNE 30th,
WE ASSUME YOU CANNOT BE WITH US.
If you wish to contact me, my office phone number [illegible]
If I am not available please direct all questions or gi[illegible]
all information to my secretary, Patricia [illegible]

Most Sincerely,

Over the years, I had received a "golf ball" type invitation to Roy's golf outing.

Drug companies are in business to make money. Not one drug company exists only to help people who need pharmaceuticals. Certainly, drug companies have human individuals in their business who like to play golf, or swim, or anything completely unrelated to the manufacture and production of pills and capsules – but basically, every drug company exists to make money.

Yes, millions of dollars worth of drugs have been given to foreign countries where thousands of sick people cannot receive proper help and certain drugs are a real necessity. I personally have been involved in working with Mylan Pharmaceutical Company as a corporate board member to supply millions of dollars worth of drugs to a number of poor countries that have minimal access to these medicines.

1965 – JAMAICA

It's always nice to have friends, particularly if these are golfing friends. Burt Gookin, a friend for many years, was president of H.J. Heinz Company and of course had the use of the Heinz plane. In 1965, Burt invited my wife and me to accompany him and his wife on a flight to Jamaica to play golf. We accepted. It just so happened that I had a personal connection with the Children's Hospital in Jamaica, having aided in the training of one of their young doctors in pediatric surgery.

My discussions with this young surgeon revealed how serious the financial situation was at his Children's Institution. I made a rather prompt decision as to what I was going to do with a rather large amount of money that I controlled in a rather peculiar fashion. It had happened that some years previously I had performed operations on a child to repair a congenital cleft lip and palate, and the family of this child had no money even to pay for the hospitalization.

"Someone" anonymously contacted me about that congenital lip/palate and arranged for me to use the $50,000, which the "someone" was offering for surgical care of similar medical problems. However, for some strange reason, I could not legally use this money in the United States and, of course, it was not for my personal use.

I made contact with the young surgeon who had trained with me, and I arranged to meet him at his hospital in Jamaica. Visiting that hospital was an enlightening experience – it needed financial help and I could legally turn that money over to that institution. The $50,000 made available to that hospital was just a drop in the bucket to what was needed, but without a doubt, it was really put to good use.

Back to golf in Jamaica! Burt had a very good friend, Bob Wegeman, from Syracuse, New York. Bob had a beautiful home in Jamaica, not too far from the airport, on top of a hill overlooking a beautiful golf course. The golf course was Tryall Golf Club – and Bob Wegeman owned that course.

Obviously, we were comfortable at that golf area as we were all staying at Bob's house. However, while the golf course was superb, playing conditions were somewhat unique. Because of the numerous robberies in Jamaica, Bob had unusual protection for us to be able to rest without very much concern about invasion of the house or during play. Bob had numerous men carrying rifles protecting all of us in his home. And when we played golf, these men with rifles on their shoulders were with us on every hole that we played. This was the only golf experience that I ever had under such conditions – but an unbelievable golf setup.

One last notation regarding Burt Gookin and Bob Wegeman – they talked golf, played golf, and were rather reluctant to discuss any kind of business. Later, after returning to Pittsburgh, I learned that Burt and Bob were deeply involved in the invention and development of the scanner, that little flat glassed-in-apparatus that prices all of our food in the grocery store. Both had millions of dollars – all from the food business?

12 || SURGERY & BUSINESS (HOME CARE)

Surgery and business continue to work as close partners in the performing of errors in the management of each specialty. As a surgeon, I feel that we surgeons have many more opportunities than other types of medical personnel to overlook numerous important patient necessities. The surgeon advises his patient on the changing of his surgical dressings at home, taking the proper medicines with regularity, and ensuring a return to the surgeon on the day given to him.

But, the surgeon too often fails to discuss types of home care with his patient that has nothing in any way to do with surgical incisions or casts. I am one of those surgeons who for untold years failed to recognize the importance of "general home care."

It just happens that currently I have been extremely fortunate in obtaining extensive information regarding a former hospital surgical patient who lives at home and demands complete physical care. Previously I had known a former hard-working registered nurse, Sandra (Sandy) L. Dunkel, R.N., who currently is director of a superior company, Care At Home. This company, based on Freeport Road near Pittsburgh, Pennsylvania, maintains a superior position regarding the difficult work of complete home care.

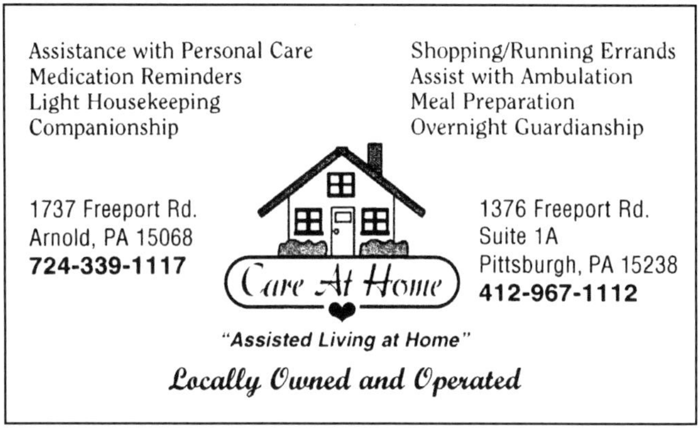

Recently, it was rather important for me to discuss the home management of a patient, so I had the opportunity to discuss the "home care" coverage work with Sandy Dunkel. Sandy was an excellent individual with whom to speak, and who did not object to my numerous, and sometimes rather dumb, questions. I learned many, many things during our talk; things that had I known years ago would have made me a much better surgeon. So – let's just listen to what Sandy said about the "home care" demands.

"It was a rude awakening when I had an uncle become terminally ill. I was working in the university/hospital setting and needed help to help him. The resources were difficult to find and when I did find them I wasn't sure what to ask or what my or his needs particularly were. All I knew for sure, was I needed someone with him when I couldn't. I had no idea where to find this person, whether I could trust them and would they treat him with the love and respect, as well as being well trained.

"The doctors would listen to my concerns and they would give me a script to obtain home care, however what I did not realize at the time, it would only cover intermittent care (short visits 10 to 30 minutes of care by a RN, PT and/or bath aide). I needed longer periods of time, I needed someone there when I couldn't be, to help getting him out of bed, assisting in the bathroom and making a meal. It just seemed that the services just did not exist.

"I learned a lot caring for my uncle those 8 months. I realized that he and I were *not* the only two that were struggling to obtain home-care. Many individuals needing home-care are concerned about costs; 'will it be too much, can I afford to have it, maybe I'll go without for awhile.' Next they know they need 'something' but what? Will the caregiver just sit around, do I have to tell them what to do, do I always have to have them.

"While I was working at the university and during my uncle's illness I started doing research on homecare. I found a family owned agency out of Philadelphia that was beginning to franchise. This company was named Special Care and I opened my own office in 1993. This became the *best* nursing I had ever done. In 2003 I became Care At Home, individually owned and operated.

"In the last 15 years there have been many gains as well as flaws in the homecare arena. There has been more availability of services throughout the state, naturally bad. Individuals are seeing that this may be a good business; forgetting that it involves individuals, ill ones at that. They are opening businesses without training, experience or support of the workers who are doing the direct care. The state is about to change some of this; licensure will soon be mandatory. This will be a major gain for the community as a whole, expectations will be required and carried out. Why should a barber have to be licensed when hair will grow back and a direct care worker not? Individuals pay a lot for services; they deserve the best!"

I have personally been extremely impressed with regard to the business that Sandy directs and have the utmost respect for the individuals in that profession. While I am very knowledgeable about what is being done by Care At Home, I asked Sandy what kind of problems she encounters and asked if she cared to discuss this subject with me.

"Finding good caregivers is probably the number one concern of all agencies. Making sure they have *all* the characteristics of an individual you would want to come into your home, let alone care for your loved one.

"Advertising, letting people know you are around. I have the most difficulty with this one. I feel that I am somehow benefiting from their misfortune and this undoubtedly may be the most difficult time in their lives. It is truly a quandary of emotions."

I asked Sandy if the hospitals in Pittsburgh had created their own home-care type groups and was told that The University of Pittsburgh Medical Center and The Allegheny Health Systems have. These hospitals were said by Sandy to have stated that they thought the problem of home-care was "a missing link." Patients were being discharged sooner, but returning due to a lack of follow-through of treatment recommendations. They needed a way to keep individuals home longer and get them well.

Back to another question. I asked Sandy if retirement homes gave her any problems and don't they take care of retired individuals who live there?

“The care in these establishments are a little complicated. These communities are usually called ‘continuum of care communities’. The reason for that is because there are levels of care. Individuals can live independently, be assisted or require nursing home care. Once an individual becomes part of the community, they can receive more thorough levels of care while remaining in an environment that they know.

“Cost to be a part of these communities varies. Some communities require a ‘buy in’ fee, which is a one-time fee (similar to a cost of a home) then a monthly maintenance fee. Others may just have a monthly rental fee and additional costs for individual requests. Many of these communities will care for the individual to the very end. It is the concept of ‘aging in place.’

“As far as private agencies like myself providing service in these communities; sometimes yes and no. Many are beginning to provide their own, which is a very good way to make sure that the resident truly gets ‘continuum of care.’

“I think that nursing quality among hospital nurses now is far lower than when I was in nursing years ago. Today, 75% of people working in hospitals are administrators and *not* in patient care. And the nurses now have less opportunity to see a patient, or talk with a patient, and therefore are not able to identify problems, particularly ones they may encounter at home. I try to have them learn how to spot trouble and use their instincts. ‘If you think there is a problem there usually is.’”

I asked what kind of problem she has or if she has a problem, getting the right kind of workers in her company Care At Home, and how does she get them?

“It’s frustrating getting help. It does not seem proper to advertise and it really does not seem that to advertise would be comfortable. We let it be known, in a kind of talking way that we are a business that exists to help people and we are not just in business to make money. We try to get the caregiver that wants to make a difference, likes people and would rather be helping than anything else. We like our work, I personally am just glad that I'm doing what I do!

"I know that we could go on talking for hours about our work on and for people but I'm going to shut up now and let you think and write about how you have observed our workers - those you have met and observed their work. Thank you so much for this good discussion."

My personal observation and evaluation of Care At Home workers has been far superior to anything that I thought I might see. They have been completely trustworthy, *always* on time to arrive, know how to promptly manage their duties, even with some being good cooks – when they are at work during meal times. They are quick to be outspoken about any physical situations and are extremely comfortable in accepting the suggestions made by those with whom they are working.

I have nothing but the very, very best to say about the work being performed by the workers of Care At Home with whom I have been in contact.

After many of these positive statements have been made by me, one may wonder how I might know a little about Care At Home work and workers. The answer is easy to make. Care At Home business personnel, and that certainly involves the Director, Sandra (Sandy) L. Dunkel, R.N., are well-known to me on a personal basis. For five years, they have been involved in taking unusually great care of my wife Franny, who is 90 years old and has major physical problems.

MEDICAL HELP, BUT NOT ALWAYS "END OF LIFE"

At the end of May, 2009, I wrote a rather complete letter to Thomas R. Russell, MD, FACS, Executive Director of the Bulletin of the American College of Surgeons. He has been doing an extremely good job at his position, particularly the monthly publication of his "From My Perspective," two-page discussions at the beginning of the journal. In addition to the informational two pages by Dr. Russell were four extremely professionally written articles including the management of end-of-life patients by surgeons and the establishment of a new surgical specialty.

This new specialty will involve the training of the physicians to properly manage the end-of-life patient. The name of this specialty is Hospice and Palliative Medicine. Currently, there is a small percentage of surgeons as members of this specialty but everything discussed regarding the end-of-life treatment appears to be proper and effective. It appears to me that many surgeons, of various specialties, will quite soon develop a sincere interest in end-of-life medical work and become members of this new specialty.

The surgeons who have been involved in some specialties would very likely have no interest in becoming involved in any way with the person who is slowly approaching the door of death. But the surgeons who are involved in the specialty where death is not uncommon must absolutely learn how to handle end-of-life.

Here is an excellent place to quote two paragraphs of the letter I wrote and sent to Dr. Russell, of the American College of Surgeons Bulletin on May 28, 2008. They are as follows:

> The February 2008 Bulletin contains five remarkable medico-surgical discussions of end-of-life care. I have read each and every word several times of each of these surgical, educational discussions concerning nearby death.
>
> As a 93-year-old retired surgeon, I just wish that I had been smart enough to have had the knowledge regarding hospice and palliative medical care and I would have used that ability for the welfare of many of my patients.

As a surgeon, I do not intend to have a reader believe that the surgeon is the only doctor who is involved with patient death. However, there are numerous surgeons who are involved in performing the types of surgery that generally do not involve serious medical or surgical problems. Prime examples are plastic surgeons, who now have generally returned from the name "Plastic and Reconstructive Surgery" to "Plastic Surgery" and where the plastic surgeon now is performing cosmetic surgery almost completely. Having been board-certified in plastic surgery, a member of the Board of Plastic Surgery, Inc., a member of that board from 1968 through 1974, and vice-chairman of that board from June 1973 through May 1974, I feel comfortable in having relative opinions.

Currently, it appears as if plastic surgery has changed from plastic and reconstructive surgery to really almost 100% cosmetic surgery, where the basic aim is to make money. Plastic surgeons are no longer interested in head and neck surgery, traumatic surgery or burn surgery.

Actually, while I was a trained plastic surgeon, my interests were not in cosmetic surgery. Personally, I was a founding member of the American Burn Association and established the extremely successful Burn/ Trauma Unit at The Western Pennsylvania Hospital in Pittsburgh. At The Western Pennsylvania Hospital, I was chairman of the Department of Surgery from 1970 to 1985. Therefore, in that variety of surgical positions, I was exposed to such a cross section of physical human problems; there were numerous cancer and traumatic situations which drew upon the ability of the physician in charge to make various decisions regarding serious problems.

However, there are periods where death may occur but not quite at that specific time. Following are just a handful of somewhat interesting personal situations.

1.) A man from Butler was a former patient of mine, having had both eyes removed because of cancer. He had a huge dog and the two were together constantly as he had a job selling newspapers in front of the town post office. The rent had to be paid. One day, he was struck over the head, robbed and brought back to Pittsburgh, put into a bed in the men's ward at Presbyterian Hospital under my care. The big dog was slipped under his bed. When there were questions about "what are we to do about this dog?" the little, but great, nurse in charge of that floor solved the problem, stating instantly "that dog will stay under that bed as long as Mr. _____ is a patient here." There was no further discussion.

2.) A 92-year-old man had received a radical neck dissection on Wednesday and was seen to be walking rather briskly on Thursday, up and down the main corridor. The nurses thought that he actually ought to remain in bed. My comment? "Let him walk; it's the best thing an old guy could do after such an extensive operation."

3.) This seventy-some-year-old was lying in bed, eyes open, but with far advanced cancer of the face and sides of the neck. There was no way he could be saved as the blood was oozing – no, faster than that – out of a carotid artery of the left neck. Nothing of any kind could be done to save that man. I sat down beside that bed, took this man's left hand in mine, put just a little pressure over the stream of blood, and kept talking with that great guy until he died. I knew that the acceptable treatment had been carried out.

4.) At times, the family of a severe cancer patient has to talk with the doctor in charge of the patient. This patient had had extensive head and neck surgery performed but was doing well. He could take nothing by mouth and a plastic tube had been put into his stomach via the outside of his stomach. The family of this man all thought that this was the perfect time to get the patient off his heavy beer drinking routine. I did not agree and convinced this family that the patient should be permitted to continue to pour his cans of beer through the outside stomach tube. I knew that the attempt to get this patient off alcohol would very likely do more harm than good.

5.) July 26, 1993, 6:00 AM – I'm called to please come over to the home of General Matthew

Ridgway as he had fallen. Matt Ridgway, the greatest general the United States ever had, was 96 years old at that time, our immediate next-door neighbor for 40 years, and my closest friend. I dashed over, ran upstairs, and Matt was lying on the floor. I pronounced him dead. Cause of death? I would like to quote Dr. Nicholson when asked the case of death of 100-year-old Senator Strom Thurmond. He died of "old age due to multiorgan failure."

EPILOGUE

Should there be a lengthy conclusion written after spelling out individual chapters relative to medicine and surgery? I really had little interest in that initially, but after recently reading the great book, *Steel My Soldiers' Hearts*, by Colonel David H. Hackworth, my thoughts were turned toward jotting down an epilogue. Colonel Hackworth's book on the Vietnam War would not appear to have any bearing on this medical book, but here is what stirred my real interests.

Colonel Hackworth thought about the little difference between the Vietnam War and the global war against terrorism that now confronts us. And, to quote Hackworth, "The second thing that came to me was that the older I get, the clearer it becomes that the fundamentals of warfare don't really change. With technology, everything just comes faster, smarter and meaner. But the basics remain the same."

And, could it not be proper today to apply wartime thinking to medical and surgical thinking?

There certainly are absolutely clear-cut basic technical similarities. First and foremost, every doctor would certainly wish to solve his patients' problems. That has been in the mind of every doctor since there was the first doctor. Then, there were rules and regulations, accepted techniques for managing pneumonia, cuts and bruises, and everything else that medically affects humans. But the medical approach to the treatment of physical problems has been changing regularly for centuries and is continuing right up to today, April 2009, as these notes are being scribbled.

People are now living many years longer and in much more comfort, following serious illnesses and accidents. This statement is true as the result of progress having been made toward better and safer medical management. And, just because many think today that better medical drugs cannot improve upon exiting ones, and surgical operations on brains, hearts and lungs that are so radically different from the accepted top-of-the-line procedures of a few years ago won't improve in every fashion, rest assured that in a number of years or possibly even months, these so-called fancy medical surgical changes still must follow really basic principles. Colonel Hackworth clearly pointed out that following proven basic principles in fighting a war is quite similar to modern day doctors clearly following proper basic principles for the obtaining of good medical results.

In 1936, having worked my way to Europe on a Cunard liner, I spent that summer in Vienna, Austria. Having become fluent in conversational German, a former Viennese doctor acquaintance obtained a position for me as an orderly at the city hospital, the Allgemeines Krankenhaus, where I became expert at handling bedpans. I worked on the ward where the great Dr. Ignacz Philipp Semmelweis (1818-1865) discovered the cause for the hospital scourge, childbed fever (puerperal fever).

Viennese women greatly preferred to deliver their babies at home because of the large number of deaths that occurred among childbearing mothers in hospitals. Dr. Semmelweis proved beyond a doubt that these deaths were the result of doctors not washing properly between deliveries and personally infecting these mothers because of germ-carrying hands.

Dr. Semmelweis went on to describe how medical students who had perfunctorily washed their hands immediately after working in the dissecting room and then examined pregnant women were the main cause of childbed fever. It was proven that Dr. Semmelweis changed this maternal mortality rate from 12.24 percent to 0.85 percent in several years. Interesting that his medical colleagues did not accept this finding. It would be most informative for everyone interested in any type of hospital infections to read this entire section regarding Dr. Semmelweis.

Basic principles? The *Pittsburgh Post Gazette* published an article on alcohol rinses in the September 29, 2002 Sunday edition. This article began by stating that an estimated 80,000 deaths occur yearly in hospitals, the result of dangerous germs being spread to patients by the unclean hands of nurses and doctors. How long does it take for this specific deadly situation to be recognized?

Now this newspaper article points out that a very quick application and hand rubbing (seconds) of an alcohol gel will greatly reduce the spreading of germs from patient to patient in the hospitals by doctors and nurses. And it was stated that maybe doctors now won't even have to scrub their hands before operations, just massage in a little alcohol gel. We have been fast learners? Please ask the doctors and nurses on various hospital floors if this material is a superior material. Answers can be interesting. Nurses call this a sham. Doctors just smile.

This does not mean that this alcohol-based hand gel material isn't good and should not be used. It just will not replace soap and water, gentle handling of tissue and plain common sense.

THE NATIONAL ENQUIRER 64

THE BEST WAY TO PREVENT THE FLU

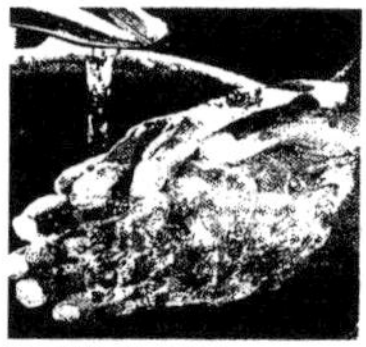

COULDN'T get a flu shot in time? Wash your hands — often!

That's your best defense against getting the flu this year, say experts.

Influenza is easily spread because it can live on surfaces for hours or days. If a person with the flu rubs his nose, then touches an elevator button, you can pick up the virus on your hand when you touch the same button.

The potentially deadly germ then enters your body if you touch your nose, mouth or eyes.

Doctors say the best way to prevent infection is simply to wash your hands before the virus can get inside you.

This small, but important, article regarding hand washing appeared in the January 2004 *National Enquirer.* It can be seen that water is running on this hand, not alcohol from a bottle. Or is this water? The article points out how one could use this technique and not bother with soap and water.

A short investigation in the West Penn Hospital Burn/Trauma Center in 2007 was interesting and somewhat educational. The short step into a room with a representative from the physical therapy department was made. As previously mentioned, each room in the Burn Center has a sink under which are foot pedals so that the hand is not necessary to turn on the water. Within three feet is an alcohol bottle on the wall.

The physical therapist demonstrated the technique, already well known to me, of striking the low end of the bottle so that alcohol would drip on the palm of his hand. And then he vigorously massaged his hands. Vigorously massaged his hands!

I made several remarks to this young man about this technique and asked several questions. First, has he noticed if everyone entering the burn room washes his hands, and whether with alcohol or soap and water, or not at all? Has he noticed the technique by various alcohol users? Ten seconds or a thorough scrubbing? And then he was somewhat shocked when I pointed out to him that he was wearing a gold wedding ring. He thought that statement was somewhat out of line as he said his wife would hill him if he ever took that ring off. He was reminded that surgeons remove rings when they operate – all of them? I then pointed out to him that millions of bacteria of any description may escape their removal by any type of hand washing, either alcohol or soap and water. And then my statement to him followed.

"Let's run a test right here in the Burn/Trauma Center to see who uses alcohol or soap and water when working in the burn room. We'll involve the pathology department and on Tuesday, January 2007, that test will begin."

The washing of hands by everyone working in hospitals is obviously unbelievably important. And recently more articles are appearing in the newspapers regarding this. The *Pittsburgh Tribune Review* on October 13, 2003 published a six-page article entitled "Hospitals Urged to Do More Against Infections," with a considerable space which covered the washing of hands by hospital personnel. This six-page discussion was followed by the same newspaper publishing a second front-page article on Sunday, October 19, 2003, with a huge front-page banner headline, "Agency (Officials of the Pennsylvania Health Care Cost Containment Council) Has Failed to Live up to its Mission."

But is all of this newspaper talk going to change the way doctors, nurses, room cleaners, engineers and administrators work toward lowering the infection rate among hospital patients? It may raise a few eyebrows.

The entire discussion of dirty hands promptly brought forth a personal experience that I could never forget. World War II ended in 1945 while I was 400 miles north of Manila near the South China Sea in a M*A*S*H unit. This unit was sent to the Japanese city of Sasebo in Kyushi for a short period before I returned to the United States. The Imperial University Hospital there needed surgical help. They had no antibiotics, minimal anesthesia coverage and no rubber gloves for surgery. I offered to work with the chief of surgery there and he taught me a lot.

This fine Japanese surgeon and I could not converse with each other, but that was a small matter. While I was already well aware of the necessity for surgeons having clean hands before operating, this experience further documented the fact that if the surgeon does the following few things absolutely properly – have meticulously clean, short fingernails, wash his hands in water using soap and extreme care, and then handle all of the organs of the patient with extreme gentility – the vast majority of post-operative problems will not be the result of infection.

STUDENTS, HOUSE STAFF, ATTENDINGS

It has been an extreme eye-opener for me to have experienced the thinking and planning of so many students, doctors, nurses, patients and others through these countless hours of discussions. Having been a medical doctor for over 60 years, shouldn't I have all the answers to most medical situations? Certainly, most physicians think we have that type of knowledge. Doctors are doctors. As stated in the Introduction, "doctors are an odd bunch of individuals as a group: the average doctor is prone to argue; he has a feeling of being somewhat important; and he is not a good listener."

But please do not forget that the basic rules and regulations of medical care. Changes will routinely occur in various ways to manage medical and surgical problems, but certain principles of care will not change. I really wished to comment somewhat on several chapters which make up this book – just plain personal thoughts as to why these individual chapter discussions were even decided upon initially and a brief summation of the "why" of these chapters.

These young men and women who are in schools of medicine and osteopathy and the medical and surgical interns and residents were unbelievably nice to converse openly with an obviously old individual. They appeared to be seriously interested in discussing the various areas that were not on their routine schedule. I was fascinated listening to various, quite personal experiences and was more than a little interested in their reactions to the variety of questions they put to me. I became educated all over again and do not wish just to make a series of discussions with this group of first-class individuals on a one-time only brief experience.

SECRETARIES

The various visits with a variety of secretaries were another worthwhile experience. Of course, without secretaries, there could be no functioning hospitals. Certainly, their work in offices and on floors has shifted in a variety of ways. The computers have eliminated so many techniques usually having been the work of secretaries that a complete description of computer/hospital functions could be written. But there remains the record work, the association of secretary with doctor and patient. The personal relationships of many years ago are noticeably different, but basic requirements of all persist.

NURSES

And then we arrive at the specialty group – nurses. Could there possibly be never-ending discussions here?

Can any hospital function without nurses? Of course not. And while we are continually hearing and reading about the acute nursing shortage, do you think for a moment that hospitals will fold and close their doors if nurses totally disappear?

Just like other serious situations have developed over the years and were acceptably solved, this is really not going to create real trouble. The problems of training, work hours, money – if the nursing shortage becomes an honestly serious situation, there will be no difficulty working out the training of nurses, arranging their working periods, and paying them the salaries they desire. Time and money never stops anything that's deemed to be absolutely mandatory.

Nurses will always be respected when they are caring for patients. There are all types of positions for nurses, but to repeat, the actual work of caring for patients is one of the most looked-up-to jobs an individual can hold. Looking back over the years of personally taking care of countless cancer patients and accident victims, I marvel at the extremely professional continuous nursing care that existed. I could never thank these many nurses for the great help they generously and continuously provided, making the medical care offered by physicians easier for the doctors and better for the patients.

But, of course, the word "doctor" had to bring forth some discussion. There has to be a page full of commentaries regarding attending physicians. Do they all think alike, believe everything they hear and read, dress in expensive and fancy clothes? In other words, do doctors all fit one mold? My answers to these questions are quite specific and likely questionable to many. It's my opinion that physicians are one of the most unusual collections of people in existence.

My respect for doctors is enormous, yet I must say that I do not agree with many decisions they make regarding non-medical business and delight in never-ending discussions on a somewhat routine basis. Doctors relish always being correct in their approach to a ruling in golf, the driving of a Ford or Lincoln car, or why the hospital administration make such a dumb decision about this new equipment.

A rather unique article appeared in the business section of the November 13, 2004 *Tribune-Review* newspaper. It stated that doctors are being urged (by whom?) to apologize and say they were sorry if they in some way made a mistake and hurt a patient. This approach, it was said, was a powerful way to soothe patients and head off malpractice lawsuits.

This article stated a frequently published report that an Institute of Medicine article in 1999 stated that medical mistakes kill as many as 98,000 Americans every year. This is a lot. But this article specifically suggested ways for doctors to handle their medical errors and was, in my opinion, just dumb. Doctors must manage their medical errors in an honest, proper fashion. And there are honest, proper ways to take care of these medical errors.

In my opinion this all goes toward making doctors quite acceptable individuals. A non-physician has little concept about our somewhat vainglorious actions. Would it not be quite an unusual surprise for you to listen to the conversation among a group of various specialty doctors at lunch some day? Your understanding of a physician as you know him may be transformed somewhat. You may come away from the lunchroom having a different slant on doctors (even a better view of them?). You will see that these doctors are honest, sincere folk who unwind somewhat when they can, talk baseball or ski trips, and have a variety of discussions. I've even heard a good joke at lunch. Just today, I had a rather lengthy discussion about several rules of golf with a noted cardiac physician, who, incidentally, is chairman of the green committee of a well-known Pittsburgh golf club, and we got into it rather heavily. Obviously, I was right and he was wrong. This candid approach could be compared to the song by the interesting singer, Mac Davis. "It's Hard to be Humble When You're Perfect in Every Way." Physicians are a breed of their own. Mac Davis's statement about being humble has been used throughout this book, and it is worth repeating.

LAWYERS

Certainly, the legal profession is frequently discussed when doctors are sorting out answers to various medical problems. Does malpractice trouble enter into these confabs? Of course. And don't we hear about malpractice cases with some regularity? The answer to that again is "yes," but with a minimum of effort, it will be shown that the newspapers and television presentations demonstrate that only the unusual and unacceptable malpractice problems are published because that's what the public wants to read and hear. What about the vast majority of physicians who adequately go about their work to have no fear of malpractice experience? A description of their work would not draw interest by comparison.

But doctors must know a considerable amount about medical malpractice. And this does not mean that they understand the legal problems that can evolve as a result of mistakes and bad luck outcomes from patient care. They must understand that good reasonable, honest patient care will void the worry and concerns that too many doctors have.

Certainly, there are lawyers who rely on medical malpractice problems for their financial income, but we all know those physicians who have had an astounding number of legal problems, and which cases are not just tough luck outcome problems, but due to the undertaking of medical problems for which they are inadequately trained or have accepted because of the rather excessive financial rewards.

Lawyers work with doctors in a variety of ways to assist us. They help us in arriving at good decisions in countless way. One of the most quieting experiences that a doctor can have is to develop a man-to-man relationship with a lawyer who thoroughly understands medical malpractice work and can comfortably discuss on a one-to-one basis. Doctors need lawyers!

DRUG COMPANIES

The newspapers are completely filled with the pharmaceutical problems that involve patients, mostly senior citizens. It will be quite interesting as to how the national government will decide. The government involvement is never ending.

Hopefully, readers may have a clearer understanding about drug companies – brand companies and generic companies. And also, there now could be those who are more interested in drug research and the unbelievable costs in that aspect of drug work.

In addition, possibly one may give some thought to buying drugs from foreign countries, including Canada. This is with the knowledge that these drugs can be dangerous, but cheaper than those that are developed in the United States.

But are all drugs that are manufactured in the United States safe? Foreign drug makers have been criticized extensively for making and selling unsafe drugs, but following is a brief resume of some American drug company experiences.

A brief article, "FDA to Revamp Drug Manufacturing Rules," appeared in the *Pittsburgh Tribune Review* of August 22, 2002. This bit of information specifically names a number of big drug companies involved, but it will suffice just to describe the problems in this discussion. The FDA admitted that it was unable to inspect drug manufactories as rigorously as it once did but would improve upon this obviously serious situation promptly.

The FDA stated the following criticisms of brand drug companies. First, it ordered a tissue bank to recall soft tissue grafts because it couldn't guarantee they were free of bacterial contamination. Next, a huge drug company agreed to a $500 million FDA fine for quality control violations. Another nationally known drug firm stated that factory problems could delay as many as five drugs under FDA review. And still another very well-known brand name drug company in 1999 paid a $100 million fine in agreeing to clean up its plants.

Certainly, every type of business has its basic problems, and the drug business definitely is no stranger to problems. Having briefly discussed this open information with several very knowledgeable friends, I was not at all surprised at how extremely surprised they were to hear openly about a subject they had never dreamed about before.

PHARMACISTS

Having grown up in my family where my dad developed and ran a drug store beginning about 1905, I obviously was exposed to drug store comments early in life. And this was an educational experience, having looked back upon those years, knowing absolutely nothing about what a drugstore (pharmacy) actually represented.

But the many and varied problems facing those managing drugs for patients today are never ending. The tremendous difference among various groups involved with pharmaceuticals is astounding. And then, the pharmacist in a small country town, the pharmacist in any area of the city, and the pharmacist in the hospital – each one has never-ending, individually important, and serious decisions to make.

It has never ceased to amaze me that we physicians have put such minimal importance on the writing of prescriptions for our patients, in and out of the hospital. My interview with the owner of the Aspinwall Pharmacy really made me reflect on the difficulties a pharmacist regularly experiences in personally providing safe and efficient care in the pharmaceutical business. The pharmacist currently fills a most important role in medical care for countless people for whom medicines are mandatory for their well being.

Are medicines dangerous for people? You can be sure that anything can happen to one under certain circumstances. Do you think that everyone is thoroughly acquainted with allergic drug reactions that can occur? That over a thousand people die every year due to their allergy to aspirin?

On Friday, September 20, 2002 in the *Pittsburgh Tribune Review*, a discussion was published regarding the inherent dangers of acetaminophen, best known by the Tylenol brand name. Acetaminophen can and does cause serious liver damage, and death can occur from the accidental taking of this drug. While acetaminophen is found in almost 200 different branded and generic products, strict attention should be paid to the label on the drug container. The FDA is just now recommending stiffer warning labels on how to use this over-the-counter drug. The FDA review found more than 56,000 emergency room visits a year due to overdoses of this drug, about a quarter of them unintentional, 100 resulting in death. Sarah Eruch, pharmacist at the University of Pennsylvania, stated that the report of 100 deaths a year was probably a severe understatement because many hospitals don't report unintentional poisonings.

So, read the labels on your medications. Do not feel bashful about discussing your drugs with your doctor and especially your pharmacist. You may be absolutely amazed at how knowledgeable your pharmacist is and how reliable and helpful he can be. Put him on your friendship list!

PATIENTS

It is quite obvious that this chapter made an attempt to specifically have doctors deal honestly with offering their patients superior care. Hospitals and the offices of doctors have shifted dramatically in the manner in which people are seen, examined and treated. Unfortunately, these changes frequently resulted in detriment to the patient.

Interestingly, it has been discussed rather extensively about the superior fashion in which patients and friends have helped their personal doctors and their hospitals. And it is not at all surprising that there are those who attempt a smile when the name Elvis Presley is mentioned. However, how many people know that the West Penn Hospital Burn/Trauma Center has received over $60,000 in donations from the We Remember Elvis Club? The Pittsburgh-based club is the largest official Elvis Presley Fan Club in the United States, with over 900 members from around the world. People sincerely want to help those who truly need help.

A rather minimal number of patient complaints about their hospitals and doctors were discussed but please believe it – there are far too many. And the majority of these complaints could easily be eliminated by sincere efforts in just the use of good common sense.

Certainly, people are aware of the shortage of nurses in hospitals, but if the hospital management is not prepared for patients to be adequately treated and cared for, such as eliminating medical errors, technical mistakes and poor bathroom care, then limit admissions and secure the satisfactory numbers and types of physicians.

Most doctors share in patient complaints? That item has been presented also. But it bears repeating. There is no possible way that doctors can expect non-doctor personnel to prevent patient accidents and complaints acceptably. This is just as much a problem for the doctors, and they must understand and accept this as a major portion of their medical practice.

It is really amazing how nurses, doctors, numerous others in hospital work, as well as patients, really enjoy the art of complaining. And this really is not all that unacceptable; it's a good kind of fun in many ways.

What really isn't funny is when nothing is done about correcting correctable problems.

This chapter on patients was the one that made me think the most about my medical experiences. It caused me to sit back and try to visualize why many patients had come to me for surgical help. Over 80 percent of my work involved head and neck tumor problems. I know that those of us who were in the head and neck cancer specialty worked diligently to properly manage those terribly complicated physical situations for our patients.

These patients trust their doctors and believe in their ability to solve their problems.

EMERGENCY ROOM

Almost everyone has, at one time or another, visited an emergency room, whether he was seeking personal medical help or assisting a friend or relative. And few can forget some or all of what was observed and experienced there.

Now there are completely trained personnel in emergency rooms, quite different from a number of years ago. For years, the various doctors on the hospital staff would be assigned to be head of the emergency room for one or two days a month. So, if the emergency room patient appeared with an apparent acute appendicitis, a psychiatrist or even a plastic surgeon may have had to decide his treatment.

There have been several references to Colonel Hackworth's book, *Steel My Soldiers' Hearts*. in this book, with considerable discussion referable to burns and the West Penn Hospital Burn/Trauma Center. Although I thought that this book had been completed, there appeared the half of one page presentation in the February 2005 issue of the *Journal of the American College of Surgeons* that was rather shocking. It is apparent that this partial page had been torn from a *Surgery, Gynecology and Obstetrics* Journal, but I had not been able to date the article to obtain the complete copy.

The astounding part of this article is that it was published in 1917 in the *Journal of the American College of Surgeons*, by Dr. Elwood B. Haworth, a surgeon at the Pittsburgh Western Pennsylvania Hospital. He had been treating burns with a paraffin preparation in 1917, a substance being used in Pittsburgh hospitals in the 1940s, and its use in various ways remains under discussion by several burn groups at the present time.

And would it not be reasonable to equate Colonel Haworth's statement from the second paragraph of this Epilogue that "the older I got the clearer it became that the fundamentals of warfare [and does that not also include medicine and surgery?] don't really change. With technology everything just becomes faster, smarter and meaner. But the basics remain the same."

THE TREATMENT OF BURNS AND GRANULATING SURFACES WITH PARAFFIN–FILM PREPARATIONS

By ELWOOD B. HAWORTH, M.D. F.A.C.S., Pittsburgh
Surgeon Western Pennsylvania Hospital

THE wax or paraffin-film treatment of burns and granulating wounds sprang from the sensational accounts of the secret French preparation "ambrine" much used in the war now going on. American surgeons returning from the war in France have given glowing accounts of the wonderful results from the use of ambrine. This led to two or three American products being placed on the market. All have followed the French example of keeping the formula a secret. It is one of the disadvantages of secrecy that we do not know what attempts have been made to secure the best possible preparation; and in the absence of this knowledge, it is reasonable to suppose that the secret preparation is capable of modifications which might add to its improvement.

To meet the demand for a non-secret ethical preparation, quite an investigation of the subject has been made by Dr. Torald Sollman which is described in an article on the subject, entitled "Suggested Formulas for Paraffin Films," which appears in the *Journal of the American Medical Association* for April 7, of this year, some extracts of which I have incorporated in this paper.

The treatment of burns and granulating wound surfaces with paraffin preparations has proved to be a distinct advance in surgery and any surgeon who has employed this method of treatment cannot but realize that the results obtained are much superior to those obtained by any other procedure.

Wounds cicatrize in one-third to one-half the time. The scar tissue is less dense and more flexible, and skin grafting is comparatively not often required. Should skin grafting be thought advisable it will be found that, under the paraffin-film application, these grafts will develop much more rapidly than by any other known method.

The action of the paraffin-film application

1917

and now, please turn this page

Surg, Gynecol & Obstet 1917;25:558

558 SURGERY, GYNECOLOGY AND OBSTETRICS

place, and we have recently adopted this rule in handling fracture cases. However, if a second operation to remove the band can be eliminated, if we can overcome the disadvantage of irritation and possible non-union by using a negligible bulk of metal—just a band of thin, strong wire—the gain is obvious.

The use of wire is not new, but the methods used have been found mechanically inefficient. The hose manufacturers and the packers and balers of various goods (from hay to old newspapers) have used wire-banding instruments. The instrument which came nearest to meeting our needs was the wire-twister used to fasten rubber hose to metal ends and joints. While this instrument most effectively answers the purpose for which it was designed, it has proved inadequate for wiring fractures; for such a twister leaves a V below the twist that impairs the fixation of rigid objects.

Our problem, therefore, was, first, to eliminate the V, and second, to secure tension without snapping the wire, and we have succeeded in making a twister which fulfills both requirements. The instrument shown will twist wire down *flat* to the bone surface. The wire can be twisted one and one-half turns after reaching the point of actual fixation.

We use phosphor-bronze wire, silvered (although that is probably entirely unnecessary), of gauge 18 to 20, Brown & Sharpe.

One wire does the work of a Parham band in most cases. Two wires will do more than any Parham band possibly can, and will leave an incomparably smaller cross section of metal about the bone.

Although the method has been used clinically in a few cases, it cannot be said to have been proved out clinically, as yet. It has worked well so far.

Its application as a substitute for the Parham band is fully justified.

Just how much can be done in the fixation of fractures by wire passed through drill holes and brought taut by this instrument, is still an open question, although it has worked well on the few cases in which we have used it.

The instrument devised has been presented before the Boston Surgical Society, and we wish to present it in print so that others may use it and judge as to its practicability.

THE TREATMENT OF BURNS AND GRANULATING SURFACES WITH PARAFFIN-FILM PREPARATIONS

By ELWOOD B. HAWORTH, M.D. F.A.C.S., Pittsburgh
Surgeon Western Pennsylvania Hospital

THE wax or paraffin-film treatment of burns and granulating wounds sprang from the sensational accounts of the secret French preparation "ambrine" much used in the war now going on. American surgeons returning from the war in France have given glowing accounts of the wonderful results from the use of ambrine. This led to two or three American products being placed on the market. All have followed the French example of keeping the formula a secret. It is one of the disadvantages of secrecy that we do not know what attempts have been made to secure the best possible preparation; and in the absence of this knowledge, it is reasonable to suppose that the secret preparation is capable of modifications which might add to its improvement.

To meet the demand for a non-secret ethical preparation, quite an investigation of the subject has been made by Dr. Torald Sollman which is described in an article on the subject, entitled "Suggested Formulas for Paraffin Films," which appears in the *Journal of the American Medical Association* for April 7, of this year, some extracts of which I have incorporated in this paper.

The treatment of burns and granulating wound surfaces with paraffin preparations has proved to be a distinct advance in surgery and any surgeon who has employed this method of treatment cannot but realize that the results obtained are much superior to those obtained by any other procedure.

Wounds cicatrize in one-third to one-half the time. The scar tissue is less dense and more flexible, and skin grafting is comparatively not often required. Should skin grafting be thought advisable it will be found that, under the paraffin-film application, these grafts will develop much more rapidly than by any other known method.

The action of the paraffin-film application

June 24, 2008

Here is the Complete article on Burns by Dr. Haworth, back at West Penn in 1917.

HERE IS THE COMPLETE ARTICLE ON BURNS BY DR. HAWORTH, BACK AT WEST PENN IN 1917.

upon granulations is largely mechanical. On cooling, the film contracts and exerts a suction action, thus inducing an active hyperæmia. By keeping the wound airtight, and by acting as a splint or scaffolding to the granulations, it promotes active proliferation of the newly formed tissue cells.

Many formulas or combinations of paraffin with other substances have been suggested and used in this country as well as abroad. All the preparations, including ambrine, have paraffin as a base and Dr. Sollman in his experiments with paraffin mixtures used 28 different ingredients including petrolatum, Venice turpentine, Japan wax, olive oil, yellow beeswax, castor oil, spermaceti, resin, cocoa butter, liquid paraffin, and the different varieties of asphalt. As compared with ambrine (which he states contains 96 per cent of paraffin) he could note no marked differences as between any of the above combinations. The different varieties of paraffin on the market have melting points varying from 48° to 53° C. and the various commercial brands differ in their physical properties, such as melting point, hardness, and flexibility. It was found that samples melting close to 50°C. are to be preferred. Aside from melting point, flexibility seems to be one of the most important features.

Most paraffins found on the market are too hard to use without incorporating some softer substance to modify and make them more flexible. The admixture of wax and resin with paraffin seems to modify it suitably for the purpose of a film dressing and Dr. Max Kahn, biochemist of the Western Pennsylvania Hospital, has suggested that 2 or 3 per cent of paraffin oil added to melted paraffin renders it much softer and much less liable to crumble upon cooling.

Dr. A. J. Hull, of the Royal Army Medical Corps, states that treating paraffin with superheated steam seems to change its character in that it becomes softer and more flexible. He also states that the results attained with its use as a dressing in burns seem indistinguishable from those of ambrine. He further states that even better results are obtained by the addition of certain antiseptics and stimulating substances. The wounds become clean more rapidly, pain decreases, and the offensive smell associated with ambrine dressings is avoided. The formula we first began using at the Western Pennsylvania Hospital was composed of 70 per cent of Gulf wax paraffin, 20 per cent of white beeswax (U. S. P.), and 10 per cent of resin.

With this product we could obtain all the effects of ambrine, but it was not so flexible and had a marked tendency to crumble. To obviate this, Dr. Kahn suggested adding 2 per cent of Russian mineral oil to the formula. Further experiments showed that the addition of a small quantity of resorcin seemed to obviate the offensive smell before referred to as following the use of ambrine.

It was then thought that the addition of some substance to the formula to promote the more rapid proliferation of the epithelial cells would prove a benefit. We have used two substances for this purpose: scarlet red and sudan III, suggested by Dr. Kahn. Sudan III seems preferable as its action as a stimulant of epithelialization is found to be more pronounced. Sudan III is a diazo compound of the aniline series, having the composition C^{22} H^{16} N^{4} O. It is soluble in alcohol, chloroform, xylol, and essential oils.

Upon the injection of certain dyes like sudan III, or scarlet red, pathologists have observed a certain stimulation in the proliferation of epithelium. This active proliferation has been ascribed by Fischer to an attraction for the epithelial cells. He called the dye, therefore, an "attraxin." The changes are primarily in the connective tissue and resemble the changes produced by chronic inflammation. When sudan III or scarlet red is injected immediately below the epithelium, the connective tissue first loses its reaction to acid dyes. Following this the epithelium begins to proliferate. The epithelial proliferation is confined to the area in which the connective tissue has undergone its modified reaction to acid dyes. The epithelium retains its normal characters, but the mitotic figures may be observed and pearl formation is common. The epithelium does not invade regions where preliminary changes in connective tissue have not occurred. The results obtained by sudan III administration are similar to the effects produced by X-rays, except that in the latter instance the epithelial cells have a tendency to invade (after a time) regions where the tissue is still normal, and thus metastases may be formed as in all malignant neoplasms (Wohlbach, Hertzler).

The formula of the wax preparation we have been using at the Western Pennsylvania Hospital for the last four or five months and from which we have attained most excellent results consists as follows:

Paraffin (Gulf Refining Co., Pittsburgh)	70.0	gm.
Liquid petrolatum, U. S. P. (paraffin oil)	3.0	ccm.
White beeswax, U. S. P.	10.0	gm.
Resin	7.0	gm.
Resorcin	0.2	gm.
Sudan III	0.05	gm.
Alcohol (95 per cent)	10.0	ccm.

The paraffin and the oil are melted in a casserole over asbestos board, the direct fire being used. The resorcin and sudan III are dissolved in the alcohol, and added drop by drop to the melted paraffin with constant stirring. The mixture is now heated until all the alcohol is evaporated. The beeswax is stirred in until melted, heat being used if necessary. Then the resin is added and mixed in thoroughly while the casserole is being heated. The mixture can be poured into molds and cooled.

Do not melt the resin by itself over a hot fire, as high organic acids of a very irritating character are produced which occasion pain to the patient and irritation to the wound. Subsequently the wax cakes should always be remelted in a *double* boiler, for if the boiler containing the wax be placed immediately over the fire, or hot plate, some decomposition of the resin in the mixed formula may take place with all the objectionable results mentioned.

TECHNIQUE OF APPLICATION

After melting the wax preparation in a double boiler it is usually applied in one of three ways:

1. Directly, with a suitable brush;
2. Sprayed on with a spraying device (like an atomizer), the instrument being kept at the proper temperature by an electric coil surrounding the parts containing the wax;
3. Saturating gauze strips, or pieces of sheet cotton, with the melted wax preparation and immediately applying the same to the surfaces to be covered. Sheet cotton, specially prepared for the purpose, has been placed on the market under the name of redintol and is very well adapted for the purpose. After the first layer of wax is applied, by one of the above methods, a piece of gauze or thin layer of cotton is placed over this application, and this is again painted with wax so that the gauze or cotton is firmly embedded in the wax. Some loose cotton is now applied over this and the part bandaged.

When the wounds are very painful or sensitive, and it is not practicable to apply the first layer with a brush, the wax may be applied by one or another of the methods mentioned. Incorporating a layer of gauze or cotton between the two layers of wax enables one to remove the whole dressing in one piece when desired.

When severe burns of recent occurrence are to be dressed, it is well to puncture all blebs and remove all loose dead skin that can be done without giving added suffering, before applying the wax dressing. At the next dressing, it will be found that quite an amount of serum has collected beneath the wax. This should be gently mopped away with cotton sponges together with the removal of all necrotic tissue. Before reapplying the wax it is necessary to dry the surfaces with hot air; otherwise the wax will not stick to the surface. This can be done with an electric hair drier commonly used by hair dressers.

To get the best results burns should be redressed daily. The gentle cleansing of the eroded surfaces, as well as the surrounding skin, of all discharge and necrotic tissue is important. This is probably best accomplished with the cotton sponge saturated with ether, being careful not to rub the granulating surfaces. Here let me say that you should also be careful that no flame be near at hand. An electric hot plate is to be highly recommended for heating the wax.

After the wax is melted in the double boiler, it should be cooled to 120° F. when it may be applied with little discomfort. An ordinary thermometer, placed in the boiler containing the wax, will serve as a guide. After some experience the dresser may not require the use of the thermometer to determine the proper temperature. By applying a film of melted wax on the back of the gloved hand the dresser can obtain a good idea of the temperature from the rapidity with which the wax solidifies and also by the heat tactile sensation of the hand. However, we have yet to see any burns resulting from applying melted wax from the double boiler.

It is certainly wonderful what comfort the properly applied wax dressing affords to patients suffering from painful burns, and it is still more wonderful to note the rapidity with which the healing process proceeds.

Although it requires considerable time to cleanse properly the burned areas preparatory to renewing the dressings, this cannot outweigh the advantages, such as the comfort it affords the patient, the shortening of the period of convalescence, the rapid promotion of epithelialization and the lessened tendency to dense scar formation.

With reference to the paraffin film there may be improvements; at present it is probably the most important addition to surgery in the treatment of burns and granulating surfaces.

REFERENCES

FISCHER. Muenchen. med. Wchnschr., 1916, liii, 2041.
HERTZLER. Treatise on Tumors, 1912, p. 44.
Ibid, J. Am. M. Ass., 1908, l, 425.
Ibid, 1910, lv, 2290.
HULL, A. J. Brit. M. J., 1917.
SOLLMAN, TORALD. J. Am. M. Ass., 1917, Nov. 14.

ABOUT THE AUTHOR

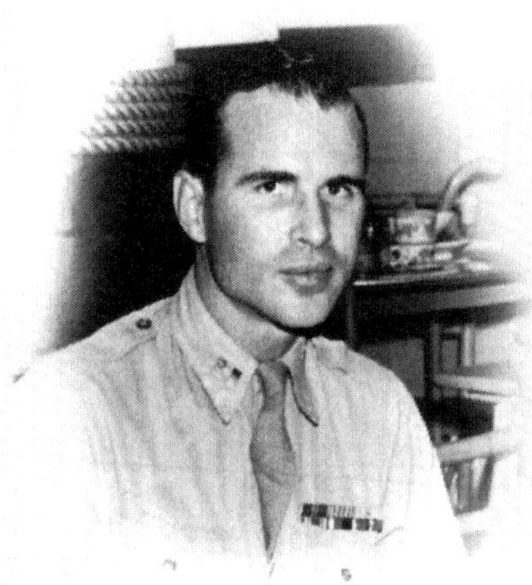

JOHN GAISFORD RETURNING HOME FROM WORLD WAR II ON THE 4TH OF JULY, 1946.

John Collyer Gaisford, MD FACS, is a retired surgeon and burn research specialist from Pittsburgh. His long and distinguished career began at Georgetown Medical School in the 1930s and then as assistant chief of surgery and chief of anesthesiology for the 92nd Field Hospital from 4 January to 3 July 1945. He was also spun off from the 92nd Field Hospital as Chief of Surgery of a M*A*S*H Unit and was sent 500 miles north of Manilla, next to the South China Sea. He ultimately received the Bronze Star for his service to the country.

Dr. Gaisford served as chairman of the Department of Surgery at Western Pennsylvania Hospital from 1970 through 1984 and founded the hospital's Burn Trauma Center in 1970. He acted as director of burn research for that center.

He was on the board of the American College of Surgeons for nine years and was its vice president for one year. He also served as president of the Ohio Valley Plastic Surgery Society (1959-63) and the Pittsburgh Surgical Society (1971). He was a founding member of the American Burn association and of the Society of Head and Neck Surgeons, of which he was also president.

He traveled the world extensively, sharing his expertise in places as far away as Suriname and Israel. He also golfed extensively, making many important and life-changing connections on the golf course.

Dr. Gaisford makes his home in Fox Chapel with his wife, Franny. They have three daughters. He has been widely published in medical journals and is the author of a biography of his famous next-door neighbor, Gen. Matthew Ridgeway, simply called *"Matt" Ridgway*, as well as *The 92nd Field Hospital: A Surgeon's Memories of WWII.* This is his third book.

WA